OSCE Skills
for
Trainees in Medicine

OSCE Skills *for* Trainees in Medicine

A Clinical Exam Guide for Students in the Health Professions

Augustine Efedaye Ohwovoriole

authorHOUSE®

AuthorHouse™ UK
1663 Liberty Drive
Bloomington, IN 47403 USA
www.authorhouse.co.uk
Phone: 0800.197.4150

© 2018 Augustine Efedaye Ohwovoriole. All rights reserved.

No part of this book may be reproduced, stored in a retrieval system, or transmitted by any means without the written permission of the author.

Published by AuthorHouse 07/18/2018

ISBN: 978-1-5462-9406-1 (sc)
ISBN: 978-1-5462-9414-6 (e)

Print information available on the last page.

Any people depicted in stock imagery provided by Getty Images are models, and such images are being used for illustrative purposes only.
Certain stock imagery © Getty Images.

This book is printed on acid-free paper.

Because of the dynamic nature of the Internet, any web addresses or links contained in this book may have changed since publication and may no longer be valid. The views expressed in this work are solely those of the author and do not necessarily reflect the views of the publisher, and the publisher hereby disclaims any responsibility for them.

To The Ohwovoriole Royal Dynasty, a Coterie of Teachers

Assessment Drives Learning

Contents

Preface xii

Acknowledgement xv

Chapter 1   Assessment of Trainee Competence in Medicine 1

Chapter 2   Overview of Objective Structured Clinical Examination 9

Chapter 3   History - taking Skills Station 29

Chapter 4   Communication and Ethics Station 59

Chapter 5   Physical Examination Skills Station 93

Chapter 6   Practical Procedure Skills Station 137

Chapter 7   Objective Structured Practical Examination 163

Chapter 8   Written or Static Station 179

Chapter 9   Structured Viva Voce Station 197

Chapter 10 Practical Assessment of Clinical Examination Skills 221

Glossary of Medical Education Terms 239

Bibliography and Resources 249

Index 255

Tables and Illustrations

FIGURES

Figure 1.1. Tools for Assessing Clinical Competencies Based on Miller's Pyramid.

Figure 2.1. Basic Schema of an OSCE Circuit.

Figure 2.2. Factors that May Impact on the Assessment of the Clinical Performance of a Candidate.

Figure 3.1. Seating Positions During History-taking.

Figure 4.1. Verbal and Non-verbal Forms of Communication.

Figure 4.2. The Face as the Mirror of the Mind.

Figure 5.1. Physical Examination Diagnostics.

Figure 5.2. Positioning of a Clinician when Performing a Physical Examination.

Figure 6.1. A Variety of Instruments and Devices May Be Placed at a Practical Procedure Station.

Figure 7.1. A Schema of an OSPE Circuit.

Figure 7.2. Potential Test Materials at OSPE Stations.

Figure 8.2. Images and Other Test Materials that Might be at Written Stations.

Figure 8.3. Chest X-ray of Yobu at Presentation

Figure 8.4. ECG Tracing of Thomas Cole

Figure 9.1. A Viva Voce Setting.

Figure 9.2. Materials and Themes for a Structured Oral Examination.

Figure 10.1. Schema of Practical Assessment of Clinical Examination Skills.

TABLES

Table 1.1. Cognitive Levels in Bloom's Taxonomy

Table 1.2. Assessment Tools by Competencies and Domains

Table 2.1. Types of Encounters or Stations in OSCE

Table 2.2. A Rating Scale for Assessing a History on Vomiting

Table 2. 3. Characteristics of OSCE Stations

Table 3.1. An Assessment Guide for a History of Abdominal Pain

Table 4.1 Essential Steps in the Process of Clinical Communication

Table 4.2. Some Popular Communication Skills Models

Table 4.3. Assessing Communication Skills at Breaking Bad News (for Postgraduates): *

Table 5.1. Positioning Doctor and Patient for a Physical Examination

Table 5.2. Assessment of Physical Examination of the Abdomen

Table 6.1. Rating Scale Assessment for Blood Pressure Measurement

Table 7.1. Features of OSPE Stations

Table 7. 2. Scoring an Experiment Station: Analytic Determination

Table 7.3. A Checklist for Measuring Blood Pressure

Table 9.1. Merits and Drawbacks of Traditional Orals

Table 9. 2. Marksheet for Structured Viva Voce Station XXIII

Table 10.1. PACES Structure and Activities

Table 10.2. Comparing PACES and OSCE

Table 10.3. Assessment Criteria for History Taking Skills in PACES

Table 10.4. Assessing Communication/Ethics Skills in PACES

Table 10.5. Assessment Criteria for Physical Exam Skills in PACES

Table 10.6. Scoring Criteria for Brief Consultation

PREFACE

The assessment of trainees is a key aspect of medical education as it is widely recognised that assessment drives learning. The tools of medical education and its assessment are continually changing. Trainers and trainees alike have to keep abreast of the trends. The objective structured clinical examination (OSCE) system has become more or less the modern gold standard in assessment of clinical students worldwide.

I have been very intensely involved with medical education including OSCE at both the undergraduate and postgraduate levels in the last several years. My purpose of writing this book and the sister version directed mainly toward the teachers is partly to use this experience to guide the trainee to clearly pass their OSCE and partly to assist teachers who are new to or unfamiliar with the OSCE system.

Most trainees in medicine and the allied professions of nursing, physiotherapy, pharmacy, dentistry etc. are likely to have a date with OSCE at the undergraduate, postgraduate, licensing and/or selection examinations. Yet too many students are scared of the OSCE system of assessment, a very fair and friendly exercise. Clinical trainees cannot therefore afford to be ignorant of OSCE.

The overarching ambition of every candidate is to pass their examinations. Your being successful at a clinical examination involves several factors, a very important one of which is your examination approach and technique. A good knowledge of the subject matter is necessary but not sufficient for you to present an impressive performance in the clinical examination especially when using tools of assessment like the OSCE, the objective structured practical examination (OSPE), and such other related examination formats like the Practical Assessment of Clinical Skills (PACES).

For you to do well in these performance-based exercises, you ought to have thoroughly prepared yourself and mastered the techniques. This book will guide you toward the goal of easily passing your clinical examinations. The book aims to equip you the trainee with the knowledge, skills, and attitudes/behaviours required of you to pass OSCEs and related examinations that demand exhibition of clinical competencies.

OSCE Skills has ten chapters. The first three chapters introduce the reader to the fundamentals of student assessment (especially OSCE) in medical education. The other chapters address systematically the various types of encounters (history taking, physical examination, communication etc) popularly referred to as stations in the parlance of OSCE and related exercises. Each encounter chapter stands on its own, starts with an explanation of the purpose of the type of station and then details what, in the assessment checklist, the examiners are likely to be looking for at such a station. The prerequisites of handling the station are presented. There is a generous provision of materials to aid reading and internalisation of the message being conveyed. Every chapter also contains illustrative examples and appendices including assessment objectives for a variety of presentations or clinical scenarios. Trainees will find these examples very valuable in self assessment and in preparation for their clinical examinations.

Trainees and others using this book should note that the OSCE Skills is on how the candidate should prepare for and behave during clinical and practical examinations in the settings of OSCE and/or its variants. The book is not a substitute for standard books on diagnosis or management of medical disorders. You, the candidate, must study your chosen standard texts and acquire the necessary clinical competencies through training; and then apply the techniques and advice espoused in this book to guide you to a respectable performance in the clinical and/or practical examination.

Good luck in your next OSCE encounter!

And Trainees and Trainees, please give me a feedback at efedaye@yahoo.com on how we can further improve *OSCE Skills*.

Acknowledgement

To Professor E.E. Ekenedigwe for the provision of radiological imagings; Professor M.A. Araoye, for permission to use his ECG tracings; and to my dear progenies, Dohwodese. Toketemu, Adonayen, and Akpifo, for their assistance in word processing and simulating.

1

Assessment of Trainee Competence in Medicine

1.1. Introduction

1.2. Purpose of Trainee Assessment

1.3. What To Assess in the Medical Trainee

1.4. Types of Trainee Assessment

1.5. Tools for Assessment of Competencies

1.6. Chapter One Summary

1.7. Chapter One Recap Exercises

1.8. Bibliography and Resources

1.1. INTRODUCTION

Expected Outcomes of Trainee Learning

The paramount goal of a curriculum for training in the health professions is to graduate competent and knowledgeable persons with the right attitude to practise the profession. To be satisfied that the trainee has achieved the intended and expected outcomes of student learning, the student has to be put to the test. This process is often referred to as **assessment**, more popularly known as **examination**.

Assessment may be defined in several ways but a simple one is that it is:
the systematic gathering and analysis of evidence to determine how competent a student is in the context of curricular goals.

The term assessment is derived from the Latin word *"assidere"* which means to "sit beside". "Sit beside" suggests that student learning or its outcome is observed critically at close quarters or bedside. Trainee assessment is typically performed by teachers in the discipline or related areas.

1.2. PURPOSE OF TRAINEE ASSESSMENT

The purpose of assessment in a medical training programme is multi-fold and will depend on the reason for which the assessment has been embarked upon. Trainee assessment is of benefit to all stakeholders in the training process and healthcare delivery: student (yes, trainees too!), the teachers, the university, the profession, and the public. Some of the principal reasons for embarking upon the student assessment process include the following:
- **For the Trainee**
    o To determine if a student has achieved the learning outcomes envisaged for the programme
    o To provide feedback information to the learner
    o To promote behaviour of self-reflection and self- correction
    o To promote access to advanced training
- **For the Public and the Profession**
    o To protect the public through identification of and denial to practice by inept individuals

- o To identify, classify, and certify/license competent trainee graduates to practise
- o To provide information for evaluation of a curriculum. or programme
- o To maintain professional and academic standards

1.3. WHAT TO ASSESS OF A MEDICAL TRAINEE

A training programme should have well articulated goals and objectives expressed in its curriculum detailing the intended learning outcomes for the trainees. It is the attainment of these goals, objectives, and learning outcomes that are the subject of student assessment. The standard content of assessment consists of **knowledge, skills, and attitude and behaviours**.

Competencies Suitable for Student Assessment

In the health professions, domains or competencies suitable for student assessment include but not limited to the following:
- Ability to interpret and synthesise clinical data
- Attitude and behaviours
- Communication and interpersonal skills
- Data gathering skills
- Ethics and legal aspects of the profession
- Knowledge of the specialty
- Performance of clinical procedure
- Professionalism

Bloom and Miller

BENJAMIN BLOOM'S DOMAINS OF EDUCATIONAL ACTIVITIES

Two names are closely associated with development of assessment in medical education: *Bloom and Miller*. In 1956 Benjamin Bloom identified three domains of educational activities:
(a) *cognitive*, mental skills (**Knowledge**);
(b) a*ffective*, growth in feelings or emotional areas (**Attitude**); and
(c) p*sychomotor*, manual or physical skills (**Skills**).

The cognitive or knowledge domain is most well described and applied. In the majority of cases, assessment will focus at one or more of these levels. Table 1.1 summarises the main categories of the cognitive domain of Bloom's taxonomy, which range from simple recall of facts to problem solving and judgement.

Table 1.1. Cognitive Levels in Bloom's Taxonomy

Level	Examples
KNOWLEDGE OR REMEMBERING	
Recall data or information. Remembering things	Recite a poem. Quote values of tests. Use mnemonics; define, list, name, recognise etc.
COMPREHENSION	
Understand the meaning and interpretation of instructions and problems	Explain in one's own words the steps for performing a task; interpret patient data; paraphrase a document
APPLICATION	
Using knowledge in a new situation	Use a formula to calculate, drug dosage, calorie needs
ANALYSIS	
Separate concepts into component parts for easy understanding	Troubleshoot an equipment; analyze, compare or contrast, distinguish, outline
SYNTHESIS	
Put parts together to form a whole; make a diagnosis	Problem solving; make a design, diagnose, summarise, write an essay
EVALUATION	
Make judgements about value of ideas or materials	Make a selection, decide pass or fail, justify a decision

GEORGE MILLER'S PYRAMID OF COMPETENCIES

George Miller introduced a similar concept in the clinical setting, often referred to as Miller's pyramid or triangle of competencies. Miller's triangle descrobes competencies ranging from factual knowledge (*knows*) at the base of the pyramid to professional practice (*does*) at the work place occupying the apex of the pyramid. The skills at the apex are more difficult to assesses but new tools such as the *mini-CEX* have been developed to assess these at the workplace.

1.4. CATEGORIES OF TRAINEE ASSESSMENT

Assessment may be categorised in a number of ways. Assessments may be written or performance- based. Another fundamental classification of tests is the division into *formative and summative* assessments. The difference between the two lies in the purpose of the assessment and at what stage in the training programme the assessment is undertaken.

Formative Assessment

The purpose of *formative or diagnostic assessment* is to determine how much the student can do and what their areas of strengths and weaknesses are. Feedback to trainees doing well can also help motivate them further. A formative assessment is usually undertaken within the course of the programme and not at the end; it is not usually used to determine the candidate's passing or failing the course.

Summative Assessment

Summative assessment is used to take decisions about the progress or fate of the trainee. Summative assessment is sometimes referred to as *assessment OF learning* as against formative assessment which is also referred to as *assessment FOR learning*. Summative assessment may be used by trainers to discover what a learner has achieved during the programme of study by gathering information from different sources, and should usually take place at the end of the programme or course. It often consists of multiple tests from the final examination and in-course or continuous assessment. The outcome of the summative assessment is used to determine exiting from a programme, placement, promotion, fitness to practise a profession or ranking of candidates.

1.5. TOOLS FOR ASSESSMENT OF COMPETENCIES

For an assessment to be reliable and effective, some techniques are better suited for certain skills than others. Figure 1.1 and Table 1.2 show the types of tools usually recommended for assessment of a variety of competencies. No one technique is good enough to assess all competencies. Therefore, in any given course, several tools are often used in the assessment of students especially those in the health professions, a principle referred to as *triangulation*.

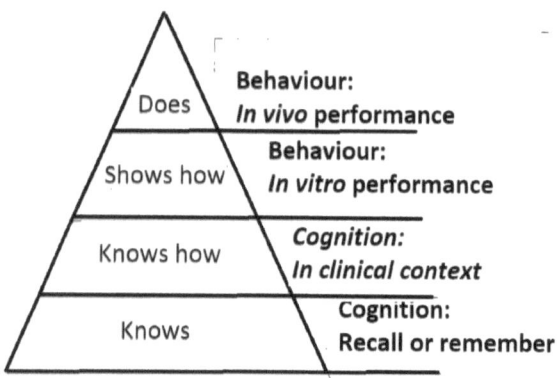

Figure 1.1. Tools for Assessing Clinical Competencies Based on Miller's Pyramid. *At the base of the pyramid are the simplest skills of remembering facts and at the apex the complex competencies of how a clinician performs in real life situation at work. The Assessment tools range from factual tests for assessment of 'knows' to in vivo techniques for assessment of what the clinician 'does' at the work place.*

The principle of *triangulation* posits that whenever possible, full assessment should be obtained from more than one source, on more than one occasion, and using more than one assessment method. Thus a comprehensive assessment may consist of marks derived from in-course tests, MCQs, essays, and clinical assessment.

1.6. CHAPTER ONE SUMMARY

Trainee assessment is the process of ascertaining whether students have achieved or are achieving intended learning outcomes. The process may involve answering questions using pen and paper (written examinations) or candidates being observed performing technical and clinical tasks (performance-based assessments). These assessments may be done in the context of *formative testing* to find out what candidates may need to improve upon or for decisions (*summative assessment*) to be taken on the candidate's progress.

Effective assessment should encompass testing at different levels in the cognitive domains and in the pyramid of competencies proposed by Miller. Trainee assessment should embrace the principle of *triangulation*.

Table 1.2. Assessment Tools by Competencies and Domains

Competency/Domain	Usage/remarks
Multiple-choice questions	
Knowledge and understanding	Summative and formative assessments
Short-answer questions	
Ability to interpret diagnostic tests; clinical reasoning	Summative and formative assessments
Structured /modified essays	
Synthesis of information, data interpretation	Mostly used in preclinical settings
Structured direct observation with checklists for ratings	
Communication skills, clinical skills	Used in clinical settings
Oral examinations	
Knowledge, clinical reasoning	Limited use except structured
Standardised patient examinations	
Some clinical skills, IPC*	Formative and summative assessments
360-degree evaluation: by peer, patient, self	
All domains	IPC* skills, professional behaviours
Assessment by patients	
Patient satisfaction; communication	Formative and summative appraisal
Assessment by peers	
Professionalism; work habits, IPC* skills, and teamwork	Formative feedback
Self-assessment	
KSA†, beliefs, behaviours	Formative and summative, reflection
Objective structured clinical examination (OSCE)	
Most domains	Formative and summative

*IPC, Interpersonal and communication, KSA† Knowledge, skills, and attitude

1.7. CHAPTER ONE RECAP EXERCISES

1. In what five ways is assessment of benefit?
2. What is the difference between formative and summative assessment?
3. Name two persons closely associated with assessment of trainees.
4. List five competencies that can be assessed in your discipline.
5. Enumerate the six levels in the cognitive domain of Bloom's taxonomy.
6. To which levels of Bloom's taxonomy do writing an open essay and answering MCQs respectively belong?
    i. What is the full name of Miller (of the Pyramid of Competencies' fame)?
    ii. What are the levels of competencies in the pyramid or triangle of Miller?
7. Justify the use and give examples of triangulation in the assessment of trainees in the health professions.

1.8. BIBLIOGRAPHY AND RESOURCES, See page 249

2

Overview of Objective Structured Clinical Examination

2.1. Introduction

2.2. Purpose of OSCE

2.3. Organisations Using OSCE

2.4. Scope of Assessable Competencies in OSCE

2.5. Categories of OSCE Stations

2.6. What Examiners Are Looking for in OSCE

2.7. Assessing Candidate Performance in OSCE

2.8. Operational Elements of an OSCE Station

2.9. Tips for the OSCE Candidate

2.10. Chapter Two Summary

2.11. Chapter Two Recap Exercises

2.12. Bibliography and Resources

2.1. INTRODUCTION

Some of the motives for the assessment of medical trainees are outlined in Chapter 1. These purposes may be summarised as: judging mastery of essential skills and knowledge; rank ordering students; measuring improvement over time; diagnosing student difficulties; providing feedback to students; evaluating the effectiveness of a course; motivating students to study; setting standards; and quality control for the public. Among the reasons and usefulness of OSCE as an assessment tool are that it:

- provides a format able to assess most components of clinical competence
- is best suited for testing clinical, technical, and practical skills
- can test across a very broad range of skills with high validity and reliability
- can test skills other common techniques cannot assess reliably e.g. communication skills
- is accepted by many medical education authorities worldwide to assess student's clinical skills
- helps to assess the effectiveness of a curriculum
- if used formatively, gives students feedback on their clinical skills
- helps to identify strengths and weaknesses in the curriculum
- helps to emphasize the importance of clinical skills in the curriculum

What is OSCE?

As mentioned elsewhere the assessment of medical trainees' competencies can be categorised in several ways such as written and performance-based forms. The **O**bjective **S**tructured Clinical **E**xamination (OSCE) is the most popular of the performance-based assessments. OSCE is a scheme of examination in the educational domain of medical and health professionals; it focuses on testing performance or more appropriately, demonstration of *'shows how'* competencies in Miller's pyramid of clinical skills rather than testing just factual knowledge.

Historical Perspective and Structure of OSCE

The **O**bjective **S**tructured **C**linical **E**xamination system was developed in Scotland by Harden and colleagues in 1975 with the purpose of rectifying some of the shortcomings associated with the traditional method of examining clinical students, *viz* using a long case and a number of short cases.

STRUCTURE OF OSCE

An OSCE exercise consists of a series of patient or problem encounters (referred to as *stations*), which a group of candidates has to rotate through within a given time, *performing the same tasks and being rated by the same examiners in the same setting using the same structured scoring scheme*. Figure 2.1. Depicts schematically the structure of an OSCE exercise.

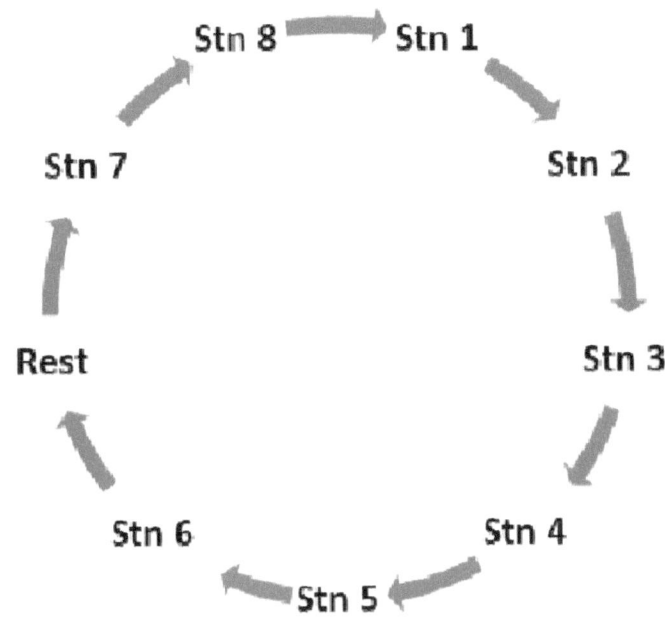

Figure 2.1. Basic Schema of an OSCE Circuit. *An OSCE circuit consists of a series of encounters termed stations (STNs). There are principally three types of station: manned stations, response or written stations and rest stations. Candidates spend the same time (usually 3 -10 minutes) at a station before moving on to the next when a signal goes.*

The number of stations in an OSCE exercise tends to vary with the discipline and/or subspecialty among other factors. The task to be performed, how the candidates should be graded, and the timing are clearly defined before the examination starts, using a structured format (*checklist or rating scale*) for scoring the candidates. A typical OSCE circuit consists of about fifteen such stations.

2.2. PURPOSE OF OSCE

The OSCE was developed to rectify the limitations associated with the traditional assessment methods of clinical skills using the long -short cases' model. The main purpose of assessing candidates should be to determine how much they know or have acquired during the training. In the examination setting, all factors except the candidate's competence should be held 'constant'. However, this is often not the case when using the traditional assessment methods; the factors of types of patient, examiner, assessment tool, and the environment can too often become serious contenders (cofounders) in determining the assessment outcome, if not controlled for.

Desirably, all the other variables in the examination setting should be held constant except the candidate's performance. In the traditional medical approach using long cases, the cases often vary in diagnosis and level of difficulty. The examiner's gradings as well the questions asked often *ex tempore* by the examiners may equally vary. The outcome of student performance, therefore, in such a traditional examination can be very dependent on the patient encounter (easy or difficult case) as well as the type of the examiner encountered -whether the candidate meets a dove or a hawk examiner, see also Figure 2.2.

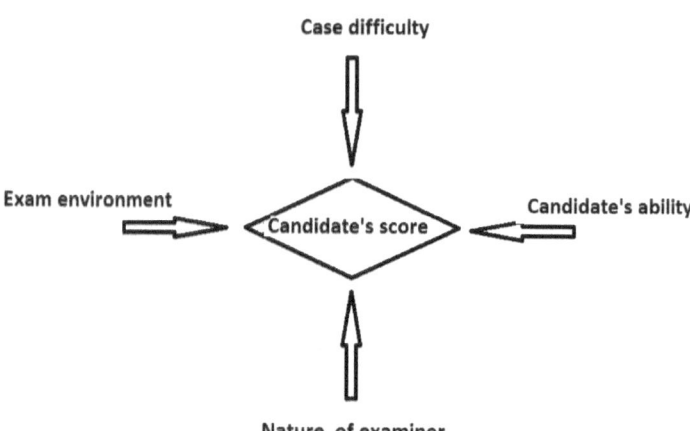

Figure 2.2. Factors that May Impact on the Assessment of the Clinical Performance of a Candidate. *Some of these factors can be controlled by the candidate who has prepared well for the exercise; some others are beyond the candidate's control. Attempts are made to control as many of these variables as possible. Using OSCE we can to a large extent control the factors emanating from the environment, patient characteristics, and the examiner.*

Harden and his colleagues introduced the objective structured clinical examination. (OSCE) removes or at least reduces several of the shortcomings in the traditional examination systems by structuring all aspects of the encounter: the patient, the marking system, and increasing the number of examiners as well as the number of clinical encounters. OSCE thus serves many useful purposes in trainee assessment and has therefore been adopted by many organisations and medical schools worldwide. It is also the choice of many a candidate.

2.3. ORGANISATIONS USING OSCE OR ITS VARIANTS

The Objective Structured Clinical Examination, since its introduction, has gained world-wide acceptance. Its use as OSCE *per se* or in a modified form has spread widely from Dundee in the UK to hundreds of countries and thousands of institutions all over the world. It was initially used only for assessment of undergraduates but it is now used in both undergraduate and postgraduate assessment across many disciplines in a variety of formats. Some of the notable organizations that use OSCE or its variants in assessment of clinical skills include the following:

- Educational Commission for Foreign Medical Graduates (ECFMG) USA
- General Medical Council of the UK
- Major Colleges of Medicine in Nigeria
- Medical Council of Canada
- Most medical schools in the UK, North America, Australia New Zealand.
- Postgraduate Medical Colleges in West and Southern Africa
- Professional and Language Assessment Board (PLAB) in the UK
- Schools of Pharmacy, Nursing, Physiotherapy and other allied health professions.
- The Federation of State Boards of Physical Therapy (USA)
- The National Board of Medical Examination (USA)
- The Royal Colleges in the UK
- United States Medical Licensing Examination (USMLE)

Variants of OSCE

Objective Structured Clinical Examination is being used by almost all the major disciplines in medicine and allied health professions, albeit in different variations. The common variants of OSCE include:

- GOSCE or TOSCE   Group (Team) objective structured clinic examination
- OSLER   Objective structured long case examination record
- OSPE   Objective structured practical Examination
- OSPRE   Objective structured performance-related examination
- OSSE   Objective Structured Selection Examination
- OSTE   Objective structured teaching evaluation
- OSVE   Objective structured video examination
- PACES   Practical assessment of clinical examination skills

OSCE or its variants may be used formatively at the beginning of and during a programme or summatively for important decision process such as selecting candidates, graduating students, granting practice licence etc.

2.4. SCOPE OF ASSESSABLE COMPETENCIES IN OSCE

Almost any skill or competency in medical education can be assessed in an OSCE exercise. Among the common OSCE-examinable skills are:

- Ability to answer short answer questions
- Communication and interpersonal skills
- Counselling
- Data interpretation
- Decision making
- Ethical and legal issues
- History taking
- Image and tracing Interpretation
- Management options
- Obtaining informed consent
- Patient education, explanation
- Physical Examination
- Presentation of clinical findings
- Problem solving
- Professional attitude
- Technical / practical procedures

The OSCE system has a lot of flexibility and practicability and can thus be adapted to assess a wide variety of competencies and application of medical knowledge. Skills and competencies suitable for assessment in OSCE include taking a clinical history, performing a physical examination, interpersonal and communication skills, attitudes and behaviours, and interpretation of data and images. In recent times performances on machines or other devices (as patient substitutes) have been incorporated into OSCE or its variants.

Key Features of OSCE

OSCE is adaptable across professional, clinical, and academic levels, with a potential for peer assessment and feedback. One particular advantage of the OSCE system is its comprehensiveness in sampling the curriculum. The key features of OSCE are summarised below and treated in greater detail in other sections of this book:

- *Structure of OSCE*
    o A number of stations/encounters arranged in a circuit focusing on performance testing
- *Purpose of OSCE*
    o Used either as a teaching tool (formatively) or a decision instrument (summatively).
- *Station purpose*
    o To test the trainee's ability to demonstrate a specified competency under observation
- *Durations of Circuit and Station*
    o A circuit consists of 8-25 stations, each station lasting 5 - 10 minutes. OSCEs for formative exercise usually contain fewer (5-10) stations
- *Movement of Examinees*
    o A set of examinees rotates through the stations in the circuit with each examinee being assessed by one or more examiners at each station.
- *Task Presentation*
    o Clinical problems at a station may be presented by a standardised or real patient; as photograph, data interpretation; or performance of a procedure.
- *Simulated Patients (Tutored Patients or Actors)*

- - Simulated patients (actors or tutored patients) in place of real patients are frequently used as persons portraying the intended disorder.
- *Scoring Instruments*
  - Examinees are rated or scored by the examiner/examiners using a previously agreed format of a marking scheme or checklist.
- *General Merits of OSCE*
  - Assessment by OSCE removes variability in patient difficulty, examiner variation, questions, and marking schemes; improves fairness to the candidates.
- *Reliability and Validity*
  - *OSCE has a high reliability* and validity as an assessment tool compared to traditional means of assessment.

Some examining bodies build into OSCE an oral examination encounter component (*viva voce*) and data interpretation as well as radiological images. All such tasks and practical tasks when integrated into a non-clinical examination, are sometimes referred to as Objective Structured **Practical** Examination (OSPE). However, the terms OSPE and OSCE are often used interchangeably.

2.5. CATEGORIES OF OSCE STATION

The *station* or *encounter* is the operational unit of the OSCE system. There can be several types of encounters or stations in OSCE depending on the purpose of the exercise. At the onset of the usage of OSCE, there were two principal stations: a *procedure or manned* station and a *post-encounter probe* station, the latter being a question station deriving from the activities in the preceding station. A third inactive station referred to as *rest station* completed the traditional OSCE stations. With wide-spread usage and modifications, the types of stations have increased, although most of the new types of stations are modifications of the initial three stations. Table 2.1 shows the common types of OSCE stations, which may broadly be classified as *manned, unmanned, clinical, practical or interactive and non-interactive.*

Table 2.1. Types of Encounters or Stations in OSCE

Station type	Description
Manned or Interactive Stations	
Clinical	Candidate interacts with patient; Examiner observes and scores; a standardised patient may also score.
Practical or technical procedure	Candidate performs a task on anatomical model, human being or mannequin etc. Examiner observes, scores and/or interacts with candidate.
Structured viva	A situation is presented to candidate. They are asked to discuss their analysis or interpretation of the issues or facts and recommend next line of action.
Couplet station	May be manned or unmanned; task at this station is linked to an immediate previous one.
Unmanned or non-interactive station	
Static or Written information	Written information or data for the candidate to interpret and answer. Answers graded later electronically or manually
Rest Station	Task-free; no examiner present; may be overseen by an assistant who attends to candidate's needs, if any. May contain water or a drink.

The number of stations in most OSCE circuits ranges from 8-25 (median about 15) of such encounters, the maximum number being partly determined by the purpose and depth of tasks and tools being used for the particular overall assessment. The task to be performed, how the candidates should be graded, and the timing are all defined for each station, using a structured format.

Interactive or Manned Stations

Manned or interactive stations are those encounters requiring the presence of examiners or raters. These are usually stations featuring clinical scenarios (history-taking, physical examination, patient education etc.) and therefore involve a real patient or often a *simulated patient* (SP). The other type of station that is manned is the "practical procedure station" at which candidates are required to demonstrate their skill at a technical procedure e.g. cardiopulmonary resuscitation (CPR) and catheterization. Simulators, models and mannequins are usually used in place of human subjects in some practical procedure skills stations.

Unmanned or Non-interactive Station

At an *unmanned (also referred to non-interactive or static station)*, the candidate is presented with information to which they are asked to respond appropriately. The questions may be based on the preceding station or new "independent" patient information, data, or imaging. Examples of common unmanned stations include writing a prescription, reading an ECG tracing, and interpreting data or radiographs. Candidates record their responses to the structured task on an answer sheet provided. Written stations may be included in the OSCE circuit or may be administered at another time and location. Examiners are not required to observe students at static stations but may be required to grade their responses.

Couplet Stations

At the couplet station, the task before the candidate is based on another (usually preceding) manned station. The couplet station may be manned or unmanned depending on the purpose and nature of the task. Thus short answer questions or MCQs may be presented at this station. On the other hand, the station may be made interactive, in which case the candidate is asked to present and/or discuss findings, management etc. of the patient encountered at a preceding station.

2.6. WHAT EXAMINERS ARE LOOKING FOR IN OSCE

The three key outcomes of medical education needed to be assessed are medical knowledge, skills, and attitude to the profession and patient care. Of these, practical skills and attitude have the pride of place in OSCE. Medical knowledge is better assessed using other assessment techniques like MCQs but a sound medical knowledge is also needed to perform well in OSCE. Some of what the examiners expect of you at an OSCE station listed below are elaborated upon in the relevant sections:

- Knowledge
  - demonstrating understanding and application of underlying basic concepts
- History-taking
  - maturely and confidently obtaining an appropriate and focused systematic history

- Physical Examination
  - maturely and confidently making an appropriate and a focused one
- Management
  - synthesising a management plan based on the differential diagnosis/problem
- Diagnosis and synthesis of data
  - Ability, maturity and confidence to collate data from history and examination, to synthesize differential diagnoses or a problem list; synthesise results of investigations (if appropriate)
- Record Keeping
  - concisely and accurately recording notes, compiling drug charts, writing referral letters and medico-legal documents
- Case Presentation
  - With maturity and confidence succinctly and coherently presenting a case using appropriate medical terminology and in a systematic manner
- Technical Procedures
  - Maturely, and confidently setting up and performing tasks appropriate for the job (e.g. functional assessment, suturing, ECG, IV cannulation, etc).
- Patient-centred Care
  - with maturity and confidence developing and maintaining a therapeutic relationship with patients and families
- Communication
  - communicating with maturity, empathy, and confidence; using non-verbal cues and successfully concluding a consultation in an appropriate manner
- Demonstrating listening, narrative and nonverbal skills
- Investigation Plan
  - Using information obtained in collating clinical data to develop an appropriate list of investigations; appreciating the necessity to follow-up any result ordered
- Organisation
  - Ability, maturity, and confidence to document key information, with focused, comprehensive reporting approach

- Ethics and the Law
  - Ability to recognise and explain the ethical dimensions of medical practice; to demonstrate an understanding of the legal demands on the medical profession
- Professionalism
  - Ability to recognise the holistic nature of professional commitment and to appreciate the changing nature of medical professionalism
- Self-Care
  - Ability to demonstrate an awareness of the principles of self-care and the importance of personal development for medical professionals
- Scope of Practice
  - Ability to demonstrate procedures related to delivering a particular aspect of clinical care based on current research and best clinical practice
- Planning
  - Ability to anticipate and plan in advance; to prioritise conflicting demands and build contingencies; demonstrate effective time management.

2.7. ASSESSING CANDIDATE PERFORMANCE IN OSCE

A candidate's performance at each station is individually scored against the criteria set forth for assessing that particular skill/exercise. The total points available for each station may vary, as well as the points needed to pass each station. A mark of "Fail" in an individual active station will not necessarily be an automatic failure for the entire OSCE as the total marks for the exercise are aggregated to determine whether a candidate passes or fails.

Grading of a candidate's performance at an OSCE station uses mainly two forms: *checklists or rating scales and grading of short answer questions*. Generally at manned stations scoring is by means of rating scales (Table 2.2) from one or more examiners while written or unmanned stations make use of short answer responses or MCQs.

Grading Candidate Performance at an OSCE Station

Table 2.2. A Rating Scale for Assessing a History on Vomiting

Activity	Satisfactory		
	Yes	No	ND
1. Introduction	2	1	0
After introduction candidate asks:			
2. When and how did vomiting start?	2	1	0
3. How many times do you vomit in a day?	2	1	0
4. Is the vomiting worse in the mornings? Is the vomiting effortless?	2	1	0
5. How is the vomiting related to meals?	2	1	0
6. How much do you vomit? Is the vomit copious and watery? Colour of the vomit?	2	1	0
7. What does the vomitus contain [Any blood, bile, or food in the vomit?]	2	1	0
8. Has the vomiting affected your weight? Any Fever?	2	1	0
9. Does he feel sick before vomiting?	2	1	0
10. Is the vomiting associated with an abdominal pain?	2	1	0
11. Does he feel better after vomiting?	2	1	0
12. Has he travelled recently?	2	1	0
13. Any other members of the family or close friends affected?	2	1	0
13. Is he taking any medications?	2	1	0
15. Is there any other association.	2	1	0
16. Does he have a history of peptic ulcer, gallstones etc.?	2	1	0
17. Is there any other information he wants to tell candidate about the vomiting?	2	1	0
18. Summarises; thanks patient; closes	2	1	0

ND, Not Done

CHECKLIST OR RATING SCALES

The *checklist or rating scale* system consists of the station task broken down into its components. For any of the objective of the components performed you are awarded appropriate marks. The rating scale will usually not be shown to you in the examination but through practice you should become familiar with what the examiners are looking for. This book and the other resources will also guide you.

The examiners have instructions to score only the items listed on the checklist and not to deviate from it; that is part of the structuring of the examination. All the candidates going through a station will be scored using only the task components listed for each station. This is certainly fairer than the traditional approach. In the subsequent chapters of this book you will be taken through the main aspects of the tasks expected of you at the common stations in an OSCE exercise.

2.8. OPERATIONAL ELEMENTS OF AN OSCE STATION

The required elements of an OSCE station will vary according to the nature of the competence to be assessed. In general you will be provided with a set of documents giving information on what the station is about and what is expected of the candidate. Some devices or equipment that are needed for the execution of the task may also be provided.

At manned stations, there will be one or more examiners. There may also be other assistants to guide and help you if the need arises. Table 2.3 summarises what are generally provided at an OSCE station.

2.9. TIPS FOR THE OSCE CANDIDATE

To do well in OSCE, there are some requisites you need besides your knowledge and skills. You need to be smart as well.

Preparing for OSCE

Know the competencies in your discipline that are commonly assessed in OSCE such as: doing a physical examination; taking and presenting a history; performing practical clinical procedures; analysing and interpreting clinical data; and communicating with patients and relatives.

1. *Repeated Practice*! To build confidence and speed, practise clinical skills on each other and on patients. Find a study partner or a group and dedicate practice time together. Download checklists and try to simulate as close as possible the "real" examination setting. Obtain constructive feedbacks (you won't improve otherwise!) and ensure you stick to the TIME ALLOTTED.
2. *Feedback.* As you practise, provide a live commentary of the steps you are taking to a colleague. Ask them to give you a feedback on your performance.

Table 2. 3. Characteristics of OSCE Stations

Equipment	Exam Staff	Documents
History Station		
Nil	Examiner(s), Standardised patient ± Timer	*Standard general elements and PIs. loose sheets
Physical Examination Station		
Exam trolley; Hand washing materials	Examiner(s) Standardised patient	*Standard general elements and PIs. Loose sheets
Clinical Practical Procedure Station		
Special equipment, depends on type of procedure or task	Examiners(s), Technician ± SP	*Standard general elements and PIs
Communication/ Patient Education Station		
Communication-specific item	Examiners(s) and SP	*Standard general elements and PIs
Written Station: Interpretation		
Data dependent: e.g. X-ray viewing box, instrument	± Technician ± Assistant)	*Standard general elements ± SAQs, loose sheets
Attitudes and Behaviours Station		
May be needed, depends on case	Examiners (s) and SP	*Standard general elements
Problem Solving and Structured Viva Voce		
Task dependent	Examiners(s) ± SP	*Standard general elements
Patient Management Station		
Depends on case	Examiners(s) ± SP	*Standard general elements
Rest Station		
± Refreshment	-	Jotters Feedback sheet

*Standard general elements *include Station construct, Candidate instructions, Examiner instructions and Checklists or Mark sheet; PIs, patient instructions; SAQs, short answer questions; SP, standardised or simulated patient*

3. As your *confidence* grows, move from using colleagues to actual patients under the supervision of your teachers.
4. *Memorize the rudiments of history of presenting complaints* or illness questions; remember to appropriately use all seven or eight dimensions of a symptom. Find an easy mnemonic for doing things in the heat of the examination.
5. *Memorize and internalise all of the Review of Systems (ROS) questions*, especially for the pulmonary, cardiac, neurological, endocrine, and gastrointestinal systems.
6. Be conversant with *common clinical procedure encounters*; these assess your ability to perform a clinical procedure, the knowledge that underlies the skill and your communication/ethics skills.
7. Develop your own or adapt a system of solving patients' problems. The CAMBRIDGE – CALGARY MODEL OF PATIENT'S PROBLEM LIST FOR CLERKING summarised below is very good for adaptation for your own use.
8. *Cambridge – Calgary model* of Patient's Problem List is useful for tackling OSCE tasks; it consists of:
    a. Exploration of Patient's Problems [MEDICAL PERSPECTIVE (DISEASE) AND PATIENT'S PERSPECTIVE (ILLNESS)]
    b. Background Information – Context (history of past illnesses, drug and allergy, family and, Personal and Social History; Review of Systems)
    c. Physical Examination (General, focused, other)
    d. Differential Diagnosis - Hypotheses (including both disease and illness issues)
    e. Plan of Management (Investigations and Treatment alternatives)
    f. Explanation and Planning with Patient (What the patient has been told and plan of action agreed upon).
9. Among others, particularly practice and be proficient in the following common *consultation skills*: attentive listening, picking up cues, empathy, appropriate language; appropriate use of open and closed questions; clarification; and periodic summarizing of interview.
10. Have *plenty of sleep on the night before* the OSCE.

Dress Code

The following recommendation on dress code modified from a medical school. About the same may apply to your appearance at the OSCE.
1. Dress and behave professionally.
2. Clothes should be smart and clean. Avoid jeans, low cut tops, or mid riffs showing.
3. White coats should be worn according to individual hospital policy or as the examination organizers have directed.
4. Put on your name badge
5. Hair should be kept neat and tidy while women's long hair must be tied back
6. Jewelry should not be worn except for the following:

    - Rings: 3one single metal band. No rings with stones.
    - Earrings: small studs only
    - Necklaces: a simple chain allowed only if kept tucked inside clothing
    - No bracelets, charity wrist bands

7. Upper body: short sleeved tops or sleeves should be neatly folded to the elbow.
8. Ties should be secured during an examination.
9. Fingernails should be short and clean, for both male and female doctors.
10. Normal shoes- no trainers, slippers or open toes.
11. Men should not wear ear rings or braided hair
12. Perfumes if any should be minimal

During the OSCE
1. Write down the information that's presented to you; don't forget to get the "patient's" name and knock on the door, if there is one, before entering.
2. Having comprehended the instructions, spend a few seconds to outline on paper how you will go about the station. Recap your practice sessions. PLAN THE STATION; OTHERWISE YOU ARE PLANNING TO FAIL!

3. TALK BEFORE YOU TOUCH! Introduce and orientate the patient and yourself, find out or ascertain the patient's name; seek consent, and ask the patient how they might wish to be addressed.
4. Make sure you wash (or sanitise) your hands before and after you touch each patient or patient environment.
5. Pay attention to where you're standing when you perform an examination; start from the right side of the patient, even if you are left-handed.
6. Maintain rapport throughout. Explain briefly what each test or manoeuvre you perform is designed to do and/or why you have to ask certain (personal) questions.
7. Don't use medical jargon when you explain things to the "patient."
8. Establish an attentive, respectful and non-judgmental relationship
9. Acknowledge the patient's emotions and concerns.
10. Give a suitable closing statement before you leave the station. Finish the history as you would a real consultation. Don't stop communicating even if the bell goes to signify the end of the station. On your way out, add that "thank you element"
11. When required, give yourself time to think before you present your history or physical findings to the examiner.

Between Station Performances

You may be unsatisfied with your performance at a particular station, let this not stay in your mind as you move to the next stage. Remember there are several stations and that your fate is determined by your overall performance in the 15 or so stations, not just one station. So put any poor performance behind you and move ahead.

2.10. CHAPTER TWO SUMMARY

- *Objective structured clinical examination* (OSCE) is a performance-based system used mainly for the assessment of clinical students in the health professions.
- An OSCE exercise consists of a series of patient or problem encounters (referred to as STATIONS), which a group of candidates has to rotate through within a given time, PERFORMING THE SAME

TASKS AND BEING RATED BY THE SAME EXAMINERS IN THE SAME SETTING USING THE SAME STRUCTURED SCORING SCHEME.

- There are three main types of OSCE station: MANNED STATIONS with examiners present, WRITTEN STATIONS where the task requires just pen and paper, and a task-free encounter referred to as REST STATION.
- Besides examination staff at each station you will meet a set of information items the most important of which is the CANDIDATE INSTRUCTION that tells you what is expected of you at the station.
- Candidate performance is assessed (by the examiners) using a RATING SCALE or grading of response to SHORT-ANSWER QUESTIONS.
- The OSCE system is fair, flexible, and widely used across disciplines for both undergraduates and postgraduates in the health professions.
- To do well in OSCE, the candidate must know how the system operates, must have practised very well and become proficient in the workings and techniques of OSCE. Know and accept the rules!

2.11. CHAPTER TWO RECAP EXERCISES

1. What does the acronym OSCE stand for?
2. Name three variants of OSCE.
3. OSCE was introduced by whom, where, and in what year?
4. What is the operational unit of OSCE called?
5. Name the three main types of OSCE station.
6. Give two merits and two limitations of the use of OSCE?
7. Indicate true or false: OSCE

    a. improves reliability of student testing.
    b. is better for formative than for summative assessment.
    c. should be part of 'triangulation'

8. OSCE performs very well in assessing competencies *except in which one* of the following?

   a. attitude
   b. behaviour
   c. communicating skills
   d. *in vitro* performance
   e. *iv vivo* performance

2.12. BIBLIOGRAPHY AND RESOURCES, see page 249

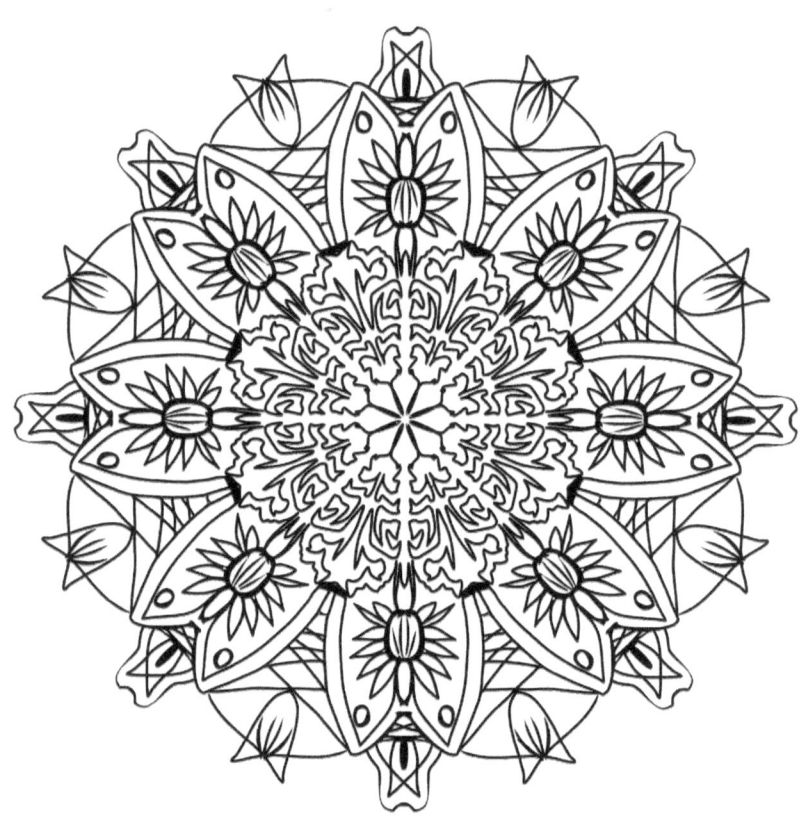

3

History - taking Skills Station

3.1. Relevance of History- taking

3.2. Purpose and Types of History Station

3.3. Staff and Essential Elements at a History- taking Station

3.4. Examiner's Expectations about Candidate's Performance

3.5. Structure and Content of the Interview

3.6. Assessable Tasks at a History-taking Station

3.7. An Example of a History-taking Station

3.8. Potential Themes for History-taking Stations

3.9. Tips on History-taking in OSCE

3.10. Chapter Three Summary

3.11. Chapter Three Recap Exercises

3.12. Bibliography and Resources

3.13. Appendices

3.1. RELEVANCE OF HISTORY-TAKING

History- taking is one of the earliest and most vital competencies a health profession trainee must acquire and would almost invariably be focused upon in any OSCE exercise, be it a formative or a summative assessment. Data gathering through history-taking probably accounts for over 70% of what is needed to make a diagnosis of most disorders. You can almost be certain that there will be one or more history- taking stations in your examination, Therefore be prepared for one or more.

There is a difference between traditional history-taking (as in a ward or clinic setting) and history-taking as applied to an OSCE setting. Given the limited time available in OSCE, it is impracticable and inefficient trying to go over the whole history with a view to covering all aspects particularly when certain areas would appear to contribute little to resolving the problem at hand. This is a common failing on the part of many a student. In OSCE, the emphasis is on a *focused history-taking* with stress on *relevant data gathering in a systematic manner*. This approach requires exhibition of your medical knowledge concerning the specific problem or case and the essentials of communication skills.

At the history-taking station, you have to explore the chief complaint/s using the history of presenting illness, past medical and surgical history, medications and allergies. In a non-emergency situation you should also obtain the details about the family and social history, occupational history, and sexual history relevant to the case scenario. Focused history-taking should not be done at the expense of missing vital information or skipping the exercise in differential diagnosis involved in exploring the history of the presenting illness.

3.2. PURPOSE AND TYPES OF HISTORY STATION

The history-taking skills station can serve several purposes such as assessment of medical knowledge, communication skills, approach to clinical data gathering, making a diagnosis or differential diagnosis, as well as problem solving and patient management. Stations may assess one or more of these skills related to the history-taking. Communication/ethics skill including professionalism is an integral aspect of a history-taking encounter and would be accorded due marks in any history-taking station involving a patient.

The type of history station will, therefore, be determined by the specific purpose or task of the station, as shown below:

- **Professionalism**
  - o To test how the candidate relates to a patient
- **Data gathering**
  - o To test candidate's ability to explore the information given by the patient with follow-up questions to reach a possible diagnosis or generate a list of differential diagnoses
- **Sensitive Information Gathering**
  - o To use an SP to collect information that ordinarily would be difficult to obtain reliably e.g. being unfaithful to a partner, being diagnosed of cancer
- **The Difficult Patient**
  - o To test how to handle the difficult, uncooperative, combative, garrulous or deceitful patient
- **Alcohol, Drug or Substance Abuse**
  - o Used to test knowledge of drug or substance abuse including alcohol and tact in obtaining such information
- **History Presentation**
  - o To systematically present information gathered in such a way as to make sense out of the available data; may be done at the same station or at a couplet or follow-up station
- **Problem Solving**
  - o Given the information obtained from the patient, to interpret the history and take decision
- **Patient Management**
  - o Given available information, to plan further management of the problem: e.g. need for examination

3.3. STAFF AND ESSENTIALS AT A HISTORY- TAKING STATION

The elements at a history station may be categorised into examination staff, documents, and miscellaneous items. For an active history-taking competency station you are likely to meet the following:

- The patient, real or often simulated (who is role-playing)

OSCE Skills for Trainees in Medicine

- Examiners, one or more; two and one being more often used at postgraduate and at undergraduate levels respectively
- Assistants for the entire OSCE or at some stations; some may act as local time minders.

The material elements at a history station will be mostly be on information describing the station and what is expected of the candidate, i.e. the task set out for the candidate. The information essentials will include *Station Title, Station Purpose, Clinical Scenario, Information and Instructions for the Candidate, Information for Simulated Patient, Information and Instructions for the Station Examiners, Checklists for scoring candidate's performance and Feedback forms.* Instructions for the patient and the examiners as well as checklists for scoring are not made available to the candidate. Besides information documents, you are likely to also have a chair for yourself. You should ask the examiners whether you may sit, before doing so (a matter of courtesy).

Candidate Briefing and Instructions

On arriving a history station, you will be given some time to read the station instructions before you interact with the patient. The instructions may also be presented to you before you enter the room. Read the instructions carefully, you may jot down the key points of the task to be performed by you. Greet both the patient and examiners before performing the history-taking. In the heat of the examination, you may forget to do these simple things, but they do count.

The candidate instruction is usually comprehensive but succinct and would include a brief description of the chief /presenting complaint/s and the setting. On the sheet containing the candidate instructions/ station briefing, you are likely to see the following information or some modification of same:

- Station Number and Station Title
- Station Purpose e.g. This station tests your ability to take a focused history from a patient who complains of cough.
- A brief description of the *Clinical Scenario*; e.g. *The patient, Mr John Part, a 55-year-old farmer, was referred to the Medical Outpatients Clinic. He complains of a cough.*

The clinical scenario may be presented separately to you or made to be part of the candidate instruction. More information might be provided such as taking notes or whether the examiners are expected to engage you in some discussion besides scoring your performance e.g. to ask you to summarise your findings to them and formulate a management plan. They may ask other specific questions as they, all the examiners, have previously agreed.

A Candidate Instructions would flow in some manner like this:

CLINICAL SCENARIO. You are a junior doctor on duty at the A&E. The patient, Mrs Amina Jumbo, is a 45-year- old woman who presents with a history of abdominal pain.

YOUR TASK: Take a focused/relevant history from the patient and attempt to make a diagnosis and/ or differential diagnoses.

TIME ALLOWED: 5 minutes

3.4. EXAMINER'S EXPECTATIONS OF CANDIDATE'S PERFORMANCE

The expectations of the examiners concerning your performance at the history-taking station may vary but would include the following essentials.

History -taking Technique

As mentioned earlier, history-taking in the OSCE setting should be different from the routine way of doing it. A comprehensive history in a regular consultation will consist of details such as the following sections:

a. Obtaining patient identifying data and the source of information.
b. Listing of the Chief Complaint/s with duration
c. History of the presenting complaint/s
d. Past medical/surgical history
e. Medications, allergies, substance use or abuse
f. Family history ± family tree
g. Personal and social history
h. Review of systems especially of the systems involved
i. Concise and clear recording of the findings

At the OSCE history station, given the limited time available and the task requested of you the candidate, the history-taking has to be *focussed and relevant* to the problem at hand. The exercise should centre on the presenting symptom/s of patient. You would be expected to:
- quickly identify the patient's personal data and the source of information.
- list the chief complaint/s with their durations.
- explore the *history of the presenting complaint* (using the eight or so dimensions) and a review of the system involved for each symptom.
- obtain a *past medical and surgical history* including medications.
- do a succinct and focussed review of the other systems.

Recording the findings may be undertaken depending on the instructions to you. Family history and social history may receive less attention at OSCE history station especially in tasks involving emergency settings. The chief complaint should receive extensive dissection that includes the following usual dimensions or attributes of any symptom:
i. Location or Site /radiation
ii. Temporal characteristics: timing (intermittent/constant), duration, and frequency
iii. The onset and setting in which the symptom occurs
iv. Quantity or intensity of the symptom
v. Quality or character of the symptom
vi. Modulating factors: relieving and aggravating factors
vii. Associated features
viii. Attributions and feelings and any prior episodes

You should have some method of remembering symptom attributes. You can use a mnemonic to aid your remembrance, such as:
- **OLD CARTS: O**nset, **L**ocation/radiation, **D**uration, **C**haracter, **A**ggravating factors, **R**eliving factors, **T**iming and **S**everity
- **SOCRATES:** Site, Onset, Character, Radiation, Associated features, Timing, Exacerbating/alleviating factors, and Severity;
- **OPQRST: O**nset, **P**alliating/Provoking factors, **Q**uality/**Q**uantity, **R**adiation, **S**ite, **T**iming/temporal relationships (duration of symptom, duration of each episode, duration of relief, frequency etc.

Identify the Chief Complaint/Entrance Complaint and fully clarify it with *the history of presenting illness (HPI)*. The purpose of the HPI is to find out how symptoms and the related events developed. The history should be an exercise in your mind on the most likely diagnoses of the complaint. The potential differential diagnosis should drive your line of questioning or focus. Try and follow the cues from the patient; do not be fixated on a particular line of reasoning. Thus if the patient says she has no cough, it is meaningless to go to ask the colour or content of sputum!

In taking the history, bear in mind the purpose of the station and what in general the examiners are expecting of you. Taking the history may follow some pattern you have established for yourself but in general be flexible while remembering that you will also be assessed both on skills in communication and knowledge of the particular task. The examiners are expecting you to demonstrate the following competencies at the history-taking station:

- COMMUNICATION SKILLS AND PROFESSIONALISM
    - Establishing rapport (initial approach and making the patient at ease)
    - Obtaining consent to conduct the interview
    - Eliciting the patient's agenda for the encounter
    - Eliciting the patient's story in their own words
    - Identifying and responding to emotional cues from the patient
    - Periodically summarizing what has been said and checking for accuracy of content and interpretation
    - Showing and verbalizing empathy
    - Usage of verbal and non-verbal communication skills
    - Appropriate use of closed and open questions
    - Creating a shared understanding of the problem
    - Demonstrating sensitivity to patient's background
    - Assuring and maintaining confidentiality
    - Negotiating and agreeing on a plan of action with the patient, a plan that includes patient and physician involvements
    - Closing the patient encounter appropriately
- KNOWLEDGE CONTENT OF THE COMPLAINT
    - Basic information about the patient
    - Description of the chief complaint
    - History of presenting illness (dimensions as appropriate)

- PREVIOUS MEDICAL HISTORY
- MEDICATIONS AND ALLERGIES
- SOCIAL HISTORY
- FAMILY HISTORY
- PERTINENT REVIEW OF THE SYSTEMS
- GENERATING AND TESTING DIAGNOSTIC HYPOTHESES

The communication/professionalism aspects at the beginning and ending of a history station are rather generic and will be common to almost all history stations. Learn how to apply them.

Recording and Reporting the History Findings

You may or may not be required to present the data gathered from history-taking. When required to do so, this may be done at the same station (with long stations as occurs with Practical Examination of Clinical Examination Skills) or at a follow-up or couplet station. It is important that you take and organise your notes for such a presentation to flow well. You may record your findings for presentation as follows:

- *In the introductory part of the records, ascertain the complaint by restating the chief* complaint with insertion of subjective comments about the patient's health at the time of the onset of the problem/symptom. The introductory sentence may include details of the past medical history if you think that the patient's illness may be directly related to an ongoing chronic disease such as a foot problem in a patient with diabetes mellitus. You should state from the onset that the patient is known to be suffering from diabetes and for what duration.
- Description of the chief complaint should form the majority of the HPI. Give the history in chronological fashion and specifically characterise the major presenting symptoms including the attributes of each complaint.
- The review of the symptoms of the body system/s relevant to the chief complaint and any risk factors should be recorded at the same time.
- A brief review of other systems that appear to have a bearing on the presenting complaint should also be undertaken at this stage. Do not try to cover all the systems, in a parrot fashion.

Whether in a comprehensive or focussed history-taking exercise, each principal complaint should be fully explored and a paragraph devoted to it in recording the history.

SOAP Technique of Recording of Findings of Clerking

A record of the interview may be conveniently summarised in the records using a problem oriented medical or health records system such as the **S**ubjective, **O**bjective, **A**ssessment, and **P**lan (SOAP) approach. The SOAP system consists of:

- **S**ubjective findings (what the patient says from exploring the chief complaint, review of the systems, etc.)
- **O**bjective findings (data obtained on physical examination and laboratory assessment); The objective data section may not fully apply at a station devoted to history-taking only except for data brought by the patient and made available to you.
- the *Assessment* section should consist of problem formulation or listing from synthesis of the available data. Such a list may be made shorter by clustering data, putting together problems that can be explained by one diagnosis.
- The *Plan* should include investigations you will order to confirm the diagnosis or rule out differentials; symptom management or recommendations on treatment, patient education, follow-up and /or referrals.

Presentation of Data Gathered

Traditionally the final aspect of the history-taking process (after performing a physical) is presentation and making sense of the data gathered. When required you should be able to present the history logically, confidently and coherently as to make sense and not just recite the facts without alluding to the positive links, offering differential diagnosis, and discussing further actions as needed. When challenged, you should be prepared to interpret the information from the history you took.

3.5. STRUCTURE AND CONTENT OF THE INTERVIEW

Besides the general technique and the communication aspects of history-taking, the interview or history-taking should also possess "substance" and "structure". You should exhibit satisfactory medical knowledge of the features and causes of the presenting complaint and its dimensions and differential. You will need to appropriately characterise the chief complaint through informed questioning. In the course of the interview, you should be able to construct a differential diagnosis list based on the information provided by the patient. Doing this will make your interview purposeful.

3.6. ASSESSABLE TASKS AT A HISTORY-TAKING STATION

The history-taking station can be used to assess several competencies as a primary aim. Secondary tasks such as communication skills and attitude as well as knowledge of medical conditions may also be assessed along with the primary competency of data gathering through history-taking. The example given in section 3.7 will help explain this further.

3.7. AN EXAMPLE OF A HISTORY-TAKING STATION

As noted earlier, the following general elements will be present at the history-taking station:
- Station title: History-taking Station
- Purpose of the Station: The purpose of this station is to test the candidate's ability to take a focused history from a patient who presents with abdominal pain and to be able give the differential diagnoses.
- Time allowed: 5 minutes
- Patient scenario
- Candidate instructions

Candidate Briefing and Instructions

SCENARIO: You are a junior doctor on duty at the A&E of a general hospital. The patient, Mrs Amina Okoro, is a 45-year- old woman who presents with a history of abdominal pain.

YOUR TASK: To take a focused and relevant history from Mrs Amina Okoro and attempt to make a diagnosis and/ or differential diagnoses.
TIME ALLOWED: 5 minutes

HISTORY - TAKING STATION

Simulated History for the Patient. *(This information will not be available to the candidate, except for the short description of the clinical scenario). The patient is schooled on how to consistently present the history and answer relevant questions from the candidates as in the following:*

YOUR COMPLAINTS

You are Mrs Amina Okoro a 45-year-old history teacher at a secondary school in this town. You came to the emergency department of the hospital this morning because of a sudden pain in the upper part of your stomach. This pain started about ten hours ago. The doctors have examined you. They have also performed some tests, the results of which are being awaited. In the meantime you have been given an injection to relieve the pain. You now feel better but are still experiencing some degree of pain.

The candidate who is a trainee doctor will ask you some questions about this pain. The details of how you should relate to the candidate are in the briefing written for you by the examiners and elaborated upon during your training sessions.

A stimulated full briefing is attached as Appendix 3.1.

Information for the Station Examiner (*This information is **not** to be made available to the candidate).*

Please read all the information pertaining to this station as well as your own instructions and the marking scheme.

Scoring Instructions

Please complete the checklist (Table 3.1) fully, leaving no item unchecked or unrated. Besides rating the performance of the candidate on the individual task components or objectives, rate the candidate *globally* as: Outstanding (5 marks), Very good (4), Pass (3), Borderline (2), Fail (1) and Abysmal failure (0) without relating global rating to your total checklist scores for this purpose. <u>Please do the global rating before totalling your checklist scores</u>. Enter your global score before the next candidate enters the room.

Please do not prompt any candidate except as previously agreed upon by all the examiners. About 30 seconds to the bell, pose the question at the bottom of the checklist to the candidate.

Table 3.1. An Assessment Guide for a History of Abdominal Pain

Task Component / Item *[Very Good, 5; Good, 4; Average, 3; Poor, 2; Very poor, or not done, 0.]*

GENERAL COMMUNICATION SKILLS / RAPPORT BUILDING

1. Initial approach / rapport (4-3-2-1-0)
2. Listening skills: shows sensitivity to the patient's view; checks what the patient says (5-4-3-2-1-0)
3. Verbal skills: Questioning, verbal facilitation, use of language, explaining, (5-4-3-2-1-0)
4. Shows empathy and nonverbal communication (5-4 -3-2-1-0)
5. Paraphrases and summarises what the patient said (5-4-3-2-1-0)
6. Identifies patients concerns and perceptions (5-4-3-2-1-0)

STATION-RELATED CONTENT

7. Asks about patient's demographic data (2-1-0)

Determines the following about the chief complaint

8. Duration and frequency of symptom (4-3-2-1-0)
9. Location of pain. Asks patient to point. Probes about radiation of pain (4-3-2-1-0)
10. Quality/character of the abdominal pain. (4-3-2-1-0)
11. Severity of the pain (4-3-2-1-0)
12. Elaborates on onset and setting of abdominal pain (4-3-2-1-0)
13. Asks about previous episodes of abdominal pain (4-3-2-1-0)
14. Asks about relieving and aggravating factors (4-3-2-1-0)

ASSOCIATED SYMPTOMS: ENQUIRES SPECIFICALLY ABOUT

15. Fever (4-3-2-1-0)
17. Loss of weight or anorexia (4-3-2-1-0)
18. Dysphagia (4-3-2-1-0)
19. Indigestion (4-3-2-1-0)
21. Nausea, vomiting, and haematemesis (4-3-2-1-0)
22. Diarrhoea or constipation (4-3-2-1-0)
23. Melena or rectal bleeding (4-3-2-1-0)
24. Steatorrhoea (4-3-2-1-0)
25. Jaundice (4-3-2-1-0)
26. Genitourinary symptoms (4-3-2-1-0)
27. Does a focused review of systems, key aspects (4-3-2-1-0)

OTHER INFORMATION

28 Medication history: Asks about past and current medications (prescribed, OTC). Takes drug and allergy history, Specific about NSAID (4-3-2-1-0)
29 Asks about treatment so far for the abdominal pain (4-3-2-1-0)
30 Asks about past medical/surgical history, key aspects (4-3-2-1-0)
31 Asks about Gynae history, LMP, dysmenorrhoea etc. (4-3-2-1-0)
32 Asks about family and social history, key aspects including alcohol (4-3-2-1-0)

Examiner: *"Please summarise your findings and offer a differential diagnosis."*

33 Summarises key findings (5-4-3-2-1-0)
34 Offers an appropriate differential diagnosis (5-4-3-2-1-0)
35 Appropriate use of open ended and closed questions (5-4-3-2-1-0)
36 Fluent and professional approach: maturity (5-4-3-2-1-0)
37 Provides appropriate closure (5-4-3-2-1-0)
38 Total for Task Components
39 Examiner's Global Rating (*circle your rating*)

NB. Depending on the responses offered by the SP, some items in Table 3.1 may not be applicable and will thus not be scored. Be focussed and avoid asking virtually all available questions including irrelevant ones, an approach that will fetch you uninspiring marks.

3.8. POTENTIAL THEMES FOR HISTORY-TAKING STATIONS

The potential themes for history stations across disciplines are almost limitless. The following are some examples of presenting complaints that can be used at a history station:

Abdominal pain	Dyspepsia	Neonatal jaundice
Alcohol	Dysuria	Nausea
Angina	Fits / seizures	Nocturnal enuresis
Anxiety	Frequency of micturition	Palpitations
Back pain		Pelvic pain
Breast lumps	Haemoptysis	Post-coital bleeding
Breathlessness	Headaches	Post-menopausal bleeding
Calf pain (claudication)	Heart failure	
Chest pain (from DVT / PE)	Heart murmurs	Pregnancy and delivery
	Hypertension	

Constipation	Incontinence	Strangulated inguinal
Cough	Incontinence	hernia
Delayed development	Infective endocarditis	Swollen joints
Diabetic	Infertility	Tall short stature
complications	Irregular heart beats	Tiredness
Diarrhoea	Jaundice	Tremor
Difficulty in	Joint pain	Urinary retention
swallowing	Loss of consciousness	Vaginal bleeding
Dizziness	Menopause	Vaginal discharge
Double vision	Menstrual	Vomiting
(Diplopia)	irregularities	Weight gain
Dysphagia	Muscle weakness	Weight loss
Febrile convulsions	Rectal bleeding	Wheezing
Dyspareunia	Renal colic	
Impotence	Short stature	

There are several reasons why candidates perform poorly at the history-taking station. Take care to avoid the following common errors among others:

1. Failure to read the station instructions thoroughly
2. Not being focussed and asking irrelevant questions
3. Failure to listen to the patient's response and concentrating on asking a series of questions by rote rather than carefully listening to what the patient has to say and responding appropriately.
4. Poor framing of questions, poor use of open-ended questions and excessive use of closed questions
5. Failure to allow the patient enough time to express the story in their own words without excessively interrupting.
6. Inability to guide and focus the interview to obtain the pertinent factual information (especially failure to clarify the history, identify the patient's previous experience with this type of problem, and gather other medical database information related to the presenting complaint)

3.9 TIPS ON HISTORY-TAKING IN OSCE

You should be properly seated as shown in Fig 3.1

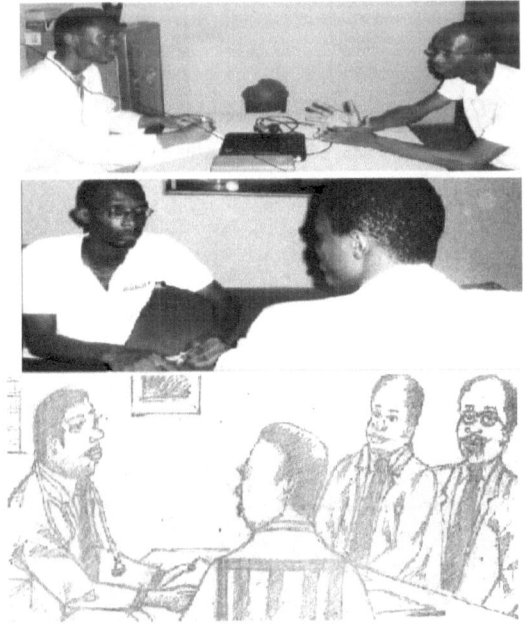

Figure 3.1. Seating Positions During History-taking. *It is not uncommon for clinicians to sit directly opposite the patient (upper panel); this position as you would with a security officer's interrogation is threatening and is to be avoided. Clinician and patient should sit at an angle in an L formation as in the middle panel. Bottom panel depicts a history taking situation with examiners present.*

7. Failure to assess the role and effect of the patient's beliefs on their illness, and their use of or belief in traditional healing/folk remedies, and/or other alternative, complementary, or integrative healing practices
8. Often, failure to briefly summarize the patient's current medical problem and its chronology, and obtain the patient's confirmation regarding the summary's accuracy;
9. It is important that you clarify the chief complaint with the history of the presenting illness. Use some mnemonics to aid your memory. Learn and follow a pattern that suits you, yet officially acceptable.

3.10. CHAPTER THREE SUMMARY

- History-taking is a vital aspect of data gathering in the work-up of the complaints of patients.
- At an OSCE history-taking station, you should exhibit professionalism (as always) and *verbal facilitation and proper use of language;* explain medical language if used.
- You should follow up on emotional cues by appropriate response to the patient's concern and anxiety.
- As the interview progresses, repeatedly paraphrase and summarise what you think the patient has said.
- Mastery of the factual content i.e. a complete description of the patient's problems is vital if you are to make some headway towards solving it.
- Communication skills are an integral part of the interview process.
- Closing or ending the encounter properly is important: *acknowledge the patient's contribution, invite any other comments or questions, and politely wind up the interview.*

3.11. CHAPTER THREE RECAP EXERCISES

1. List five competencies that can be assessed at a history-taking station.
2. List 10 objectives or task components likely to be found on the checklist at a history-taking station on dysuria.
3. Give a mnemonic for remembering the dimensions that might help you to assess a chief complaint of right lower abdominal pain due to salpingitis
4. Find out what the mnemonic CHLORIDE FPP means.
5. In summarising the history and management of a case, the SOAP technique has been found very useful. What does this acronym mean?
6. Provide three subheadings under **P** of the **SOAP** system.
7. A 36-year-old bricklayer, complains of a swelling in the right groin.
   a. Think of the differential diagnosis of this mass.
   b. Construct a checklist of about 20 items you may use to score a candidate's performance at a history station, with a particular diagnosis in mind.
8. List five common errors students often make at a history-taking station.

3.12. BIBLIOGRAPHY AND RESOURCES. See page 249

3.13. APPENDICES

Appendix 3.1. An example of a Briefing for a Simulated Patient

Introduction
This sheet summarises most of what will happen between you and the candidate. You must first read the whole story and instructions as provided in the patient profile and were told during the training. Remember to also read the instructions for the candidate and the examiner. The examiner will go over the whole scenario with you before the examiner starts. Remember to be consistent with your answers from candidate to candidate.

Simulated Patient Personal information
Name: Mrs Amina Okoro, 45 y old; Ethnicity, Duga; Religion: Muslim
You are married, have three kids; occupation, history teacher and VP. Give your address as stated. Type of housing: Three bedroom flat

1. The Problem
You came to A&E this morning with a complaint of abdominal pain. The pain started about 11 pm last night; you had attended a wedding party earlier in the day. The pain was so severe that you had to be brought into A&E instead of going to work this morning. The pain is all over the abdomen but appears to be *going to the back*. The pain started suddenly and was sharp but not colicky. The pain was of *a severity of 8 out of 10* and did not respond to anything except the injection you were given in hospital on arrival this morning. You *vomited yellowish materials* twice since the pain started. You have no diarrhoea or constipation; your stools are of normal colour and well formed. You have no fever. Your appetite has been good until the pain started last night.

You cannot understand why the pain. You wonder whether it could be due to food poison. But you ate just fried fish and had three bottles of lager beer.

2. Illnesses in the past

You have neither been admitted to hospital nor had any operation except delivery of your children usually for two days. You had a *similar pain about three years back* and was treated by the doctor with some tablets, the names of which you do not remember. That episode occurred after a naming ceremony of a friend's daughter. You vomited once that time but was not admitted. The doctor said it might have been food poison.

Specifically if asked:

Any previous operations: No.

Any previous illnesses: Occasional malaria attacks, treated with paracetamol and tablets for malaria fever.

3. Medications and allergy

Are you on any medications? *No*

Have you taken any medication taken for this problem?
No except for some Panadol® and the injection you were given today on arrival.

Contraceptive: *Not on any contraceptive*

Menses: How are your periods? *Regular, once every 28 days; lasts 3-5 days. Normal flow, no change.*

When was your last period? *Two weeks ago.*

Do you have pain before or during your menses? *No*

How old were you when you had your first menstrual period: At *age 12 years*

4. Family and Social history

Have you any family history of stomach ulcer or cancer or pancreas disuse disease? *No*

How about your parents: *father and mother alive and well*

Smoking: *Nil*

Alcohol: *Yes, details as in notes*

Social history: *Married 20 years, Children: Three, one boy, two girls.*

Occupation: *Teaching*

Husband's occupation: *Teaching*

5. Questions about any other illnesses: *answer none or as discussed.*

6. Patient's Perception of the illness (*Hypothetical exchange between Simulated Patient (SP) and Doctor, i.e. If asked, what to say*).
Doctor. What did you think might have caused this your problem?
SP. Am not sure but could be food poison at the party.
Doctor. Did anyone else at the wedding whom you know develop this type of problem?
SP. No
Doctor. What have they told you so far?
SP. Not much but Dr said we should await results of tests.
Doctor. What are you concerned about? Have you any underlying fears?
SP. I wonder if this could be ulcer or something more serious?
Doctor. What are your expectations?
SP. To find the cause of the problem and treat it once and for all.
Doctor. How are you feeling about this pain?
SP. I am anxious but feel not too bad. Just to find the cause. Not happy missing work.
Doctor. Is there anything else you need to tell me about the pain?
SP. No. Etc.

Doctor summarises what has transpired between the two and both jointly make a plan.

Appendix 3.2. A Sample of a Detailed Scoring System for a History of Abdominal Pain

The details of a history-taking as exemplified by abdominal pain might be as follow:

GENERAL COMMUNICATION SKILLS / RAPPORT BUILDING
1. Initial approach/rapport. Greets patient. Introduces self, purpose. Asks for patient's name. Seeks consent. 5=4=3=2=1=0

LISTENING SKILLS
2. Listening skills, showing sensitivity to the patient's view, checks what the patient says., Appropriate non-verbal behavior. 5=4=3=2=1=0

OSCE Skills for Trainees in Medicine

QUESTIONING SKILLS

3. Appropriate use of closed and open questions, avoids leading questions and jargons; avoids double questions; allows patient to ask questions etc... 5=4=3=2=1=0
4. Verbal facilitation: clarifies what the patients says; avoids interrupting the patient's speech. 5=4=3=2=1=0
5. Use of lay language: explaining medical language if used, avoids technical jargons. 5=4=3=2=1=0
6. Empathy expressed in words and non-verbally. Seeks patient's perception of the pain. 5=4=3=2=1=0
7. Periodically paraphrases and summarises what the patient has said. 5=4=3=2=1=0
8. Clearly identifies patient's concerns and perceptions. 5=4=3=2=1=0
9. Closing or ending: acknowledges the patients contribution, invites any other comments or questions, and politely winds up the interview. 5=4=3=2=1=0
10. Asks about patient's socio-demographics., occupation, religion etc. 5=4=3=2=1=0

CONTENT: KNOWLEDGE ABOUT ABDOMINAL PAIN SPECIFIC OBJECTIVES

11. Chief complaint: Asks about presenting complaint/s of abdominal pain and duration/s. Seeks clarification and clarifies statement. 5=4=3=2=1=0

History of Presenting illness

12. Probes location of pain. Asks patient to point. 5=4=3=2=1=0
13. Probes about radiation of pain. 5=4=3=2=1=0
14. Elaborates on onset of pain. Asks about the setting of the pain: circumstance, relation to meals or drink or other activity. Asks questions to elicit cause of pain or precipitating factors: alcohol, drugs, renal, gallbladder, cardiac. 5=4=3=2=1=0
15. Elaborates on time course of the pain: Duration of attacks, length of relief, periodicity, time course of abdominal pain. Asks about diurnal variation. Quantifies time. 5=4=3=2=1=0
16. Ascertains intensity of pain. Uses pain visual analogue or other scale as means of quantification of severity. 5=4=3=2=1=0

17. Quality/character of the abdominal pain. Asks about how the pain was like. Offers suggestions if patient appears stuck for words as to character of the pain: sharp, dull, stabbing, cramp-like, knifelike, twisting, or piercing. 5=4=3=2=1=0
18. Asks and clarifies about aggravating factors (meals, position, drugs, etc.) 5=4=3=2=1=0
19. Asks and clarifies about relieving factors (meals, position, drugs/antacids, etc.). 5=4=3=2=1=0
20. Asks and clarifies about associated symptoms (nausea, vomiting, abdominal distension, fever, vomiting, diarrhoea etc.). 5=4=3=2=1=0
21. Any other information: Asks about any other symptom or information that might be helpful. 5=4=3=2=1=0
22. Asks about PMH and especially of similar pain in the past. Specifically asks about previous history of peptic ulcer, pancreatitis, gallstones or menstrual pains. 5=4=3=2=1=0
23. Asks about previous abdominal or pelvic surgeries. 5=4=3=2=1=0

OTHER RELEVANT HISTORY

24. Focused and relevant review of systems. (symptoms that help sort out the differential and/or common conditions for patients like the one you are seeing). 5=4=3=2=1=0
25. Asks about sexual activity and history of sexually transmitted infection. 5=4=3=2=1=0
26. Family and Social History. Asks about education level, occupation and occupational exposure, travel history, marital status, children, substance abuse etc... 5=4=3=2=1=0
27. Asks about past and current medications (prescribed, OTC). Allergies. Elaborates on alcohol usage. 5=4=3=2=1=0

SUMMARY AND CLOSURE

28. Closes the interview courteously and effectively. 5=4=3=2=1=0
29. **Overall approach** (maturity, sequence, seamless transition, etc.). 5=4=3=2=1=0

30. *Answer to Examiner's Question*: Name three likely differential diagnoses of this patient's pain. One mark for each; additional point for mentioning most likely diagnosis. 4=3=2=1=0
31. *Total analytical /rating score* (out of a maximum of…)
32. *Global rating:* 5, Outstanding; 4, Clear pass; 3, Borderline;4, Fail;5, Clear Fail

Appendix 3.3. Scoring History-taking and Management Skills: Abdominal Pain (due to acute pancreatitis)

Candidate Instructions

SCENARIO: You are the Surgical JR in A&E, when Mr Joko Gbaduma a 29-year-old soldier presents with a 5-day history of vomiting and worsening epigastric pain. His vital signs are as follows: PR 98 bpm, BP 115/75 mmHg, oxygen saturation 98 per cent in air, temperature 38.5 °C and respiratory rate 20 cpm/min.
YOUR TASK: Please take a history from Mr Joko Gbaduma and form an immediate management plan.
TIME ALLOWED: 5 minutes.

Core objectives on the Examiner's Rating Scale Would Include that the Candidate

HISTORY
1. Makes appropriate introduction
2. Confirms patient's name and age
3. Establishes presenting complaint
4. Explores presenting complaint and its dimensions (SOCRATES)
5. Enquires about past medical history
6. Establishes drug and allergy history
7. Enquires about smoking and alcohol consumption
8. Closes the encounter appropriately

MANAGEMENT
9. Offers to do full examination
10. States intention to check capillary glucose

11. States intention to give analgesia Suggests taking blood for FBC and serum chemistry, LFTs, lactate dehydrogenase and aspartate transaminase, amylase, C-reactive protein (CRP), and clotting, grouping
12. States intention to cannulate, and start *i.v.* hydration
13. States intention to perform an arterial blood gas
14. Suggests a urine dipstix test and sending urine for microscopy and culture
15. States intention to request an erect chest X-ray and plain abdominal film
16. Suggests keeping the patient nil by mouth
17. States intention to prescribe compression stockings and prophylactic low molecular weight heparin
18. States intention to request an ECG
19. Suggests an ultrasound scan
20. States intention to ask for senior review

Appendix 3.4. History-taking Skills: Ectopic Pregnancy

Candidate Instructions

SCENARIO You are the HO in A&E. Mrs Iyabo Bello a 24-year-old woman complaining of severe lower abdominal pain presents. Vital Signs: temperature 38 °C, BP 125/75 mmHg, pulse rate 130 bpm, oxygen saturation 98 per cent in air.

YOUR TASK: Please take a short history and form an immediate management plan for the patient.

TIME ALLOWED: 10 minutes.

Core objectives on the Examiner's Rating Scale Would Include that the Candidate

COMMUNICATION AND PROFESSIONALISM
1. Establishes rapport (initial approach and making the patient at ease)
2. Obtains consent to conduct the interview
3. Elicits the patient's agenda for the encounter
4. Elicits the patient's story in her own words

5. Periodically summarises what has been said and checks for accuracy of content and interpretation.
6. Shows empathy
7. Uses verbal and non-verbal communication skills appropriately
8. Appropriately uses closed and open questions
9. Creates a shared understanding of the problem
10. Demonstrates sensitivity to patient's background
11. Assures and maintains confidentiality
12. Negotiates a plan of action with patient, a plan that includes patient and physician involvements
13. Closes the patient encounter appropriately

Essentials of Complaint History

14. Establishes main symptom
15. Explores symptom and asks appropriate follow-up questions
16. Enquires about past medical history
17. Establishes drug and allergy history
18. Enquires about smoking and alcohol consumption
19. Closes the interview appropriately

Management

20. Offers full examination, including a vaginal examination
21. States intention to take blood for FBC, serum chemistry, amylase, clotting screen, group and save (cross-match and rhesus status if suspected ectopic pregnancy rupture), serum save for possible beta-human chorionic gonadotrophin (_-hCG) and progesterone measurement
22. Suggests gaining *i.v.* access and commencing i.v. hydration
23. Suggests keeping patient nil by mouth
24. States intention to give analgesia and anti-emetics as required
25. States intention to request a urine dipstix test, and urinary _-hCG test
26. Suggests an urgent ultrasound scan
27. Suggests would request a senior to review

Appendix 3.5. Scoring History-taking Skills: Acute Breathlessness

Candidate Instructions

SCENARIO: You are the MO on duty when Mr Jones, an elderly gentleman, who is acutely short of breath presents to the A&E. His vital signs are as follows: temperature 37.5 °C, BP 120/80 mmHg, pulse rate 75 bpm, respiratory rate 25 breaths/min, oxygen saturation 93 per cent in 28 per cent oxygen.

YOUR TASK: Please take a history from him to enable you find the cause of the acute breathlessness.

TIME ALLOWED: 5 minutes

Core objectives on the Examiner's Rating Scale Would Include that the Candidate

COMMUNICATION AND PROFESSIONALISM
1. Establishes rapport (initial approach and making the patient at ease)
2. Obtains consent to conduct the interview
3. Elicits the patient's agenda for the encounter
4. Elicits the patient's story in his own words
5. Periodically summarises what has been said and checks for accuracy of content and interpretation.
6. Shows empathy
7. Uses verbal and non-verbal communication skills
8. Appropriately uses closed and open questions
9. Creates a shared understanding of the problem
10. Demonstrates sensitivity to patient's background
11. Assures and maintains confidentiality
12. Negotiates a plan of action with patient, a plan that includes patient and physician involvements.
13. Closes the patient encounter appropriately

ABOUT THE CHIEF COMPLAINT (ACUTE BREATHLESSNESS)
14. Establishes breathlessness as the main symptom
15. Explores the history of the presenting illness in full
16. Reviews the cardiovascular and respiratory systems
17. Asks about onset and progression

OSCE Skills for Trainees in Medicine

18. Asks about provoking and relieving factors
19. Asks about associated symptoms
20. Assesses severity of breathlessness
21. Asks about previous episodes of breathlessness
22. Asks about cigarette smoking
23. Asks about Past Medical History
24. Explores Drug history
25. Asks about Family history
26. Asks about Social history

EXAMINER: PLEASE SUMMARISE YOUR FINDINGS; OFFER A DIFFERENTIAL DIAGNOSIS

27. Summarises key findings
28. Offers an appropriate differential diagnosis

Appendix 3.6. History-taking Skills: Alcohol History

Candidate Instructions

SCENARIO: You are the registrar with the Consultant in the Psychiatry Clinic when Mrs Tresa Liman 'dragged her husband' Mr Edward Liman to see the consultant. Tresa is worried that her husband cannot stay without taking alcohol. There is a suspicion that Mr Liman is suffering ethanol dependency.

YOUR TASK: Please take a history from Mr Liman to determine his dependency status.

TIME ALLOWED: 15 minutes

Core objectives on the Examiner's Rating Scale Would Include that the Candidate

COMMUNICATION AND PROFESSIONALISM

1. Establishes rapport (initial approach and making the patient at ease)
2. Obtains consent to conduct the interview
3. Elicits the patient's agenda for the encounter
4. Elicits the patient's story in their own words
5. Periodically summarises what has been said and checks for accuracy of content and interpretation.

6. Shows empathy
7. Uses verbal and non-verbal communication skills
8. Appropriately uses closed and open questions
9. Creates a shared understanding of the problem
10. Demonstrates sensitivity to patient's background
11. Assures and maintains confidentiality
12. Negotiates a plan of action with patient, a plan that includes patient and physician involvements.
13. Closes the patient encounter appropriately

ABOUT THE HISTORY OF ETHANOL CONSUMPTION
14. Establishes alcohol intake: Amount, type/s and place

ASKS ABOUT FEATURES OF ALCOHOL DEPENDENCE:
15. Compulsion
16. Primacy
17. Stereotyped pattern
18. Increased tolerance
19. Withdrawal symptoms
20. Relief drinking
21. Asks whether patient has tried to **cut** down on alcohol
22. Asks whether patient has felt **angry** at remarks of others regarding his drinking
23. Asks whether patient has felt **guilty** about how much he drinks
24. Asks whether patient **ever drinks first thing** in the morning
25. Asks about reinstatement after abstinence
26. Asks about depression
27. Asks about common complications of alcohol misuse
28. Asks about prescribed medications
29. Asks about illicit drug use
30. Asks about family history of alcohol misuse
31. Asks about social history

OSCE Skills for Trainees in Medicine

Appendix 3.7. History-taking Skills: Depression

Candidate Instructions

SCENARIO. You are the registrar on duty in the Psychiatry Clinic with a Consultant. At the clinic is Mr Teye Tiyi, a 50-year-old engineer who says he cannot sleep and thinks that there is little to live for any more.

YOUR TASK: Talk to Mr. Tiyi in the next **TEN** minutes

Core objectives on the Examiner's Rating Scale Would Include that the Candidate

COMMUNICATION AND PROFESSIONALISM
1. Establishes rapport (initial approach and making the patient at ease)
2. Obtains consent to conduct the interview
3. Elicits the patient's agenda for the encounter
4. Elicits the patient's story in her/his own words
5. Periodically summarises what has been said and checks for accuracy of content and interpretation.
6. Shows empathy
7. Uses verbal and non-verbal communication skills
8. Appropriately uses closed and open questions
9. Creates a shared understanding of the problem
10. Demonstrates sensitivity to patient's background
11. Assures and maintains confidentiality
12. Negotiates a plan of action with patient, a plan that includes patient and physician involvements.
13. Closes the patient encounter appropriately

ABOUT THE CHIEF COMPLAINT
14. Asks about when symptom/s started
15. Explores the dimensions of the presenting complaint
16. Asks and Elicits Symptoms of Depression
17. Discusses about his mood; his feelings
18. Asks about loss of interest in pleasure (anhedonia)
19. Asks about tiredness and amount of energy (fatigue)

20. Asks about possible causes for feeling this way (bereavement stress, work etc.)
21. Asks about his hopes for the future
22. Asks about feeling of helplessness about current situation
23. Asks about how he feels about himself, his worth
24. Ask about his ability to concentrate
25. Asks about sense of guilt, who is responsible for the situation he is in.

BIOLOGICAL SYMPTOMS
26. Asks about sleep pattern (early morning waking and insomnia)
27. Asks about what time of day things are particularly bad or feels better
28. Asks about any change in appetite
29. Asks about his interest in sexual activity

DIFFERENTIALS
30. Asks about whether he sometimes feels very high and energetic
31. Asks about whether patient ever heard voices when no one else was hearing such voices etc. or seen things unusual

SUICIDAL IDEATION
32. Asks patient if he has thought of taking his own life and how often does he get such thoughts
33. Asks whether he has ever thought about ways of taking his life
34. Asks whether patient has actually attempted harming yourself and what stops him from doing it
35. Asks how have these symptoms affected his own life and that of his family

ASSOCIATED HISTORY
36. Asks about past psychiatric history
37. Asks about drug history: medications, allergies, recreational drugs
38. Asks about family history of depression or other psychiatric illness asks about employment, relationship, if he has children and support from family
39. Asks about smoking and alcohol use
40. Asks patient if he thinks he is depressed and his attitude to receiving medications (Insight)

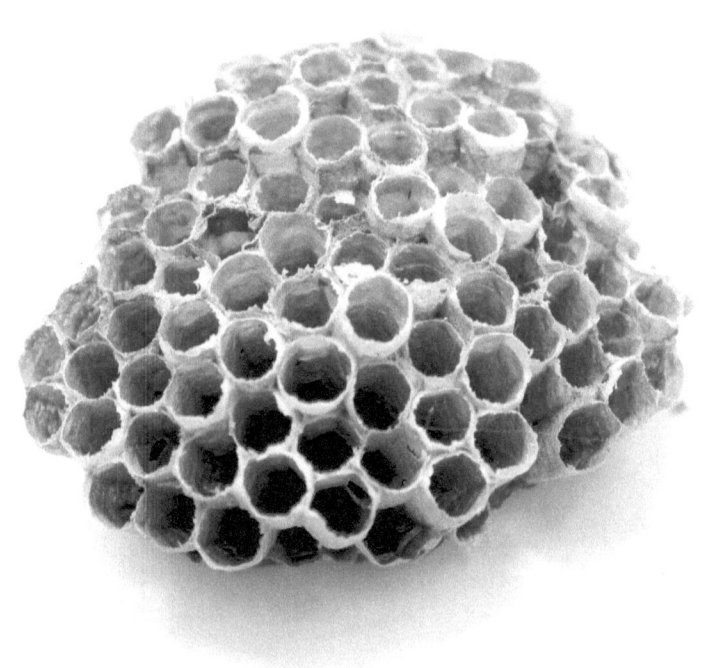

4

Communication and Ethics Station

4.1. Introduction

4.2. Categories of Communication Skills

4.3. Essential Communication Skills

4.4. Communication Skills in Clinical Context

4.5. Properties of a Communication /Ethics Skills Station

4.6. Assessment Models for Communication Skills

4. 7. Assessing Communication Skills

4. 8. Examples of a Communication/Ethics Skills Station

4.9. Advance on Handling a Communication Station

4.10. Chapter Four Summary

4.11. Chapter Four Recap Exercises

4.12. Bibliography and Resources

4.13. Appendices

4.1. INTRODUCTION

Interpersonal and communication (IPC) skills are what we use to interact or deal with others i.e. the methods we use to get our messages across to others and to comprehend the messages from them. Effective communication is a core aspect of the work of any clinician and in building and maintaining good physician-patient and physician-colleague relationships. We need effective communication in all the doctor's activities, be it history-taking, physical examination, or other encounters.

The Accreditation Council for Graduate Medical Education.(ACGME) of the United States has defined IPC as:

the ability to demonstrate interpersonal and communication skills that result in effective information exchange and teaming with patients, patients' families, and professional associates. Thus Residents (sic clinicians) are expected to:
- *create and sustain a therapeutic and ethically sound relationship with patients*
- *use effective listening skills, elicit and provide information using effective nonverbal, explanatory, questioning, and writing skills and*
- *work effectively with others as a member or leader of a healthcare team or other professional group.*

Medical ethics broadly centres on professional competence and conduct. Ethics is that branch of viewpoint dealing with rules or principles governing right conduct, values pertaining to human conduct and the moral obligation to render to the patient the best possible quality of service. Ethics also encompasses maintenance of an honest relationship with professional colleagues and the public/mankind and the consideration of the rightness and wrongness of our actions. There are four generally accepted ethical principles, viz:
- the principle of respect for autonomy (obligation to respect the decisions made by patients concerning their own lives)
- the principle of justice (obligation to treat all people equally, fairly, and impartially.)
- the principle of beneficence (obligation to bring about good in all our actions)
- the principle of nonmaleficence (obligation not to harm others: *"First, do no harm."*

The domains of medical ethics and IPC are very much intertwined in and with most of what the clinician does, You as a clinician can be effective in communicating with your patients by using plain language, listening attentively to their concerns, and encouraging patients to ask questions. Enhanced communication skills can lead to improvement in patient and physician satisfaction and in healthcare outcomes. Various forms of communication skills are required of clinicians to achieve these goals.

4.2. CATEGORIES OF COMMUNICATION SKILLS

In general, there are two main forms of communication: *verbal and non-verbal* means of communication see Fig 4.1. Verbal communication uses words to deliver the message and may be in spoken or written form. Non-verbal communication consists of expressions using body language, gestures, facial appearance, posture, and tone of voice among others.

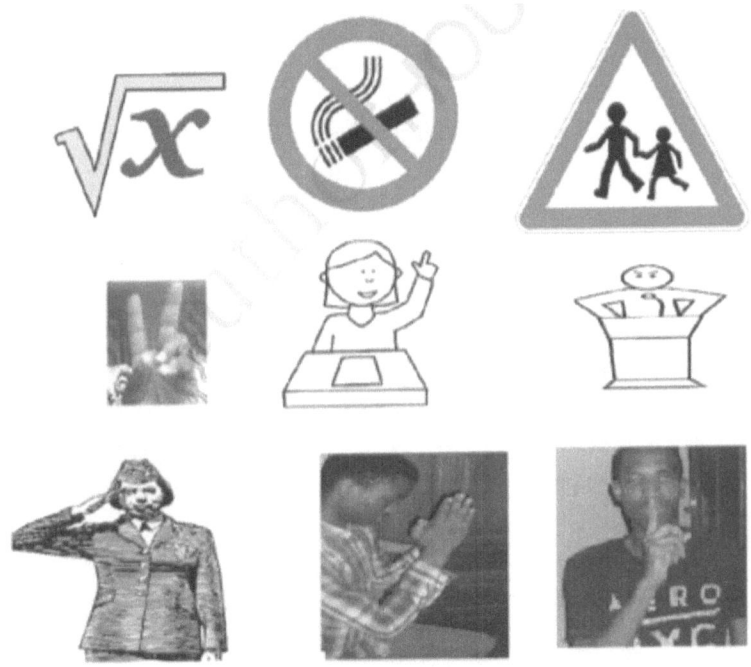

Figure 4.1. Verbal and Non-verbal Forms of Communication. *In every day life, communication can take a variety of forms from verbalising to writing and non verbal forms.*

Of the non-verbal forms of communication, eye contact and voice change are particularly relevant to the clinician. The following and Fig

4.2 show some common forms of non-verbal expressions in conveying messages:

Face: Frowning, happiness, sadness, anger and fear
Hands and fingers: Saluting, waving, pointing, and using fingers
Voice variation/ Paralinguistic: Tone of voice, loudness, inflection and pitch
Eye communication
- Direct eye contact: confidence
- Looking downwards: listening or guilty
- Single raised eye brow: doubting
- Both raised eyebrows: admiring
- Bent eyebrows: sudden focus
- Emotional tears: happy or hurt
- *Touch or haptics:* Touch can be used to communicate affection

Appearance: Choice of colour, clothing, hairstyle
Posture: Defensive postures, arm- and leg-crossing

In medicine and the allied health professions, written communication in various forms such as prescriptions and writing consults is equally important. See also section 4.9.4.

4.3. ESSENTIAL COMMUNICATION SKILLS

The three broad areas of IPC identified by *The Macy Initiative in Health Care Communication* and the seven elements of the *Kalamazoo Consensus Statement on Physician-Patient Communication* cover most of what you would need to communicate effectively with patients, their relations and professional colleagues. These skills include:

a. *The Macy Initiative in Health Care Domains of Communication Skills*
   i. Communication with the patient
   ii. Communication about the patient
   iii. Communication about medicine and science

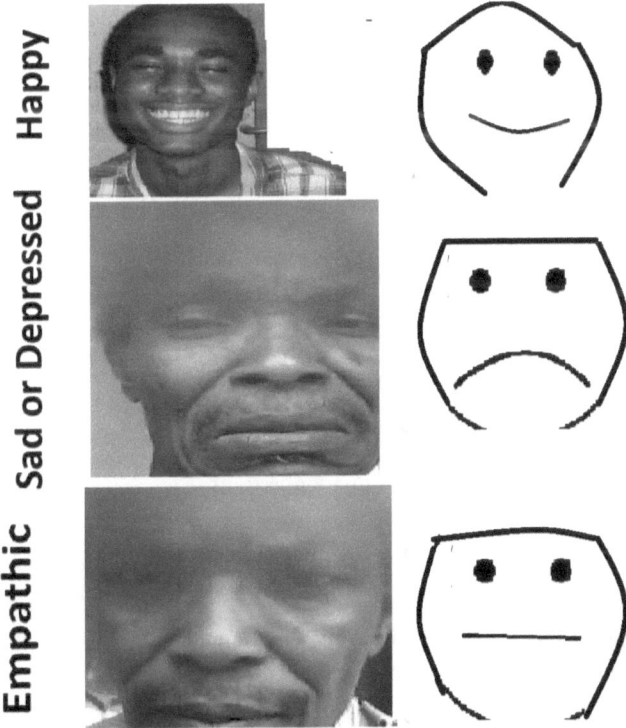

Figure 4.2. The Face as the Mirror of the Mind. *Shakespeare's famous assertion that "There's no art to find the mind's construction in the face" may not be totally correct. A lot of nonverbal communication reflecting the state of the mind or emotions can be found in the face - be it happiness, disappointment, or empathy. Note how happiness and sadness are diagrammatically represented.*

b. The Kalamazoo Consensus Statement's Seven Essential Communication Tasks

i. Build the doctor-patient relationship
ii. Open the discussion
iii. Gather information
iv. Understand the patient's perspective
v. Share information
vi. Reach agreement on problems and plans
vii. Provide closure

Table 4.1 shows in greater detail the basic elements and steps in an effective communication process in clinical context. You should learn and try to cover most of these when you are dealing with a communication theme station and in your clinical practice.

Table 4.1 Essential Steps in the Process of Clinical Communication

1. Establishing initial rapport
2. Opening discussion: Reason(s) for the consultation
3. Gathering information:
   - Appropriate use of open and closed questions
   - Exploring the problem/s
   - Verbal skills
   - Ability to explain clearly
   - Appropriate language; avoiding use of medical jargon
   - Active listening
   - Encouraging patient to ask questions
   - Non-verbal expressions
   - Summarizing and checking for understanding
4. *Exploring and understanding the patient's perspective:* *b*ackground, beliefs, values, and emotional cues
5. *Providing structure, organisation and flow*
6. *Factual content:* obtaining complete description of the patient's problems
7. Building and sustaining a *trusting relationship*
8. Sharing information and *involving the patient*
9. *Aiding* accurate recall and understanding
10. *Planning*: shared decision making
11. Pacing information and using silence
12. Demonstrating *empathy* both verbally and non-verbally
13. Maintaining rapport with the patient
14. *Reaching agreement* on problems and plans
15. Providing *appropriate closure*

4.4. COMMUNICATION SKILLS IN CLINICAL CONTEXT

As mentioned earlier interpersonal and communication skills are a very important part of clinical competencies. Besides history taking, communication skills are an integral part of the domains of attitude, ethics, and professionalism. Each of these competencies presents its own communication challenges in clinical practice. How the doctor handles the situation is important and is to be learned through practice rather than just being read from textbooks. The categories of core communication skills that trainees are most likely to encounter include the following:

a) Breaking bad news
b) Communicating with other health care professionals.
c) Communicating with third parties and relatives
d) Conducting a physical examination
e) Counselling /educating on lifestyle, health promotion or risk factors.
f) Dealing with anxious patients
g) Dealing with difficult patients and situations: the angry patient, the dying patient etc.
h) Ethical issues: e.g. confidentiality, autonomy, attitude, etc.
i) Explaining diagnosis, investigation and treatment
j) Giving instructions on discharge
k) Involving the patient in decision-making
l) Seeking informed consent
m) Taking a history or conducting a medical interview
n) Teaching a technique or a procedure
o) The angry patient, caring for the dying patient.

4.5. PROPERTIES OF A COMMUNICATION SKILLS STATION

At a communication skills station you are likely to find one or more examination staff, a patient, written instructions, and sometimes other materials and equipment.

Staff at a Communication Skills /Ethics Station

You will meet a patient (most often a simulated patient or role-player), one or two examiners, and an assistant who may also act as local time minder.

Information Items at a Communication/Ethics Skills Station

The material elements at a communication skills station would include a set of documents describing the station and what is expected of you, i.e. the task set out for the candidate. The information items usually consist of: *Station Title; Station Purpose; Clinical Scenario; Instructions for the Candidate, Simulated Patient, and the Examiners; Checklists for Scoring Candidate's Performance; and Feedback Forms.* Instructions for the patient and the examiners as well as checklists for scoring would of course not be made available to the candidate.

Information and Instructions for the Candidate

The candidate briefing is usually precise but succinct and would include a short description of the communication theme and the setting of the problem. The common *Candidate Instruction* elements consist of the following:

- Station number and Station title
- Station purpose (e.g. This station tests your ability to deliver bad news to a patient with a serious disease)
- The Clinical Scenario; e.g. *The patient, Ms Juliet Jones, a 55-year-old teacher, is being investigated for a breast mass. She has come to be told the result of the biopsy (which confirms that the growth is cancerous)*. The clinical scenario may be presented separately to you or be made part of the candidate instruction. More information may also be provided such as time limit, whether to take notes or whether the examiners are expected to engage you in some discussion. The examiners may ask you some specific questions as they, the examiners, have previously agreed.

Materials and Equipment at a Communication Station

There is likely to be a chair for you. You should ask the examiners whether you may sit. What equipment or device is presented at the Communication/ethics station would depend on the objective of the station. Stations dealing with educating patients or relatives may have things like inhalers, peak flow meters, glucometers etc. present.

4.6. ASSESSMENT MODELS FOR COMMUNICATION SKILLS

The assessment of Communication skills would follow a certain pattern depending on the theme; it may therefore be difficult to know in advance what system would be used but certain aspects are common to most communication situations. There are several models that can aid you on how you can confidently handle any communication situation. Some examples of such models are shown in Table 4.2.

Some situations such as breaking bad news or explaining /teaching a patient have their own special formats and you need to be familiar with them. The task components to be assessed vary according to the scenario and task at hand. You may find some starting blocks useful in designing your own approach. Whatever the communication skills task is, organising your approach along some or all of the elements shown in Table 4.2 would be helpful to you.

4.7. ASSESSING COMMUNICATION SKILLS

The main responsibility of the examiner or observer at the station is to rate your performance while you interact with the simulated or standardised patient (SP) in the execution of the required task. Assessing the candidate's performance at the communication station is usually done by a trainer or other professionals with some knowledge of communication skills as well as the subject matter.

The *Communication Station* feigns a consultation. You will be scored at this station on *the structure, process and outcome* of a simulated consultation, using a checklist or rating scale for the component tasks and/or global overall scale scoring system. Global assessment is done independent of the rating or checklist scores. The scoresheet may also contain, towards its end, structured questions with clear expected answers that the examiner should ask the candidate in the last few moments of the station.

Table 4.2. Some Popular Communication Skills Models

Core Communication skills

- initiating the session
- gathering information
- building the relationship
- explanation and planning
- closing the session.

The Kalamazoo Consensus Essential Elements of Communication in Medical Encounters

The GRIEV_ING Model*

G, gather; **R**, resources;, **I** identify; **E**, educate; **V**, verify; **_**, space; **I**, inquire; **N**, nuts and bolts; **G**, give

ILS model

Invite, **L**isten, and **S**ummarise

SEGUE Model

The **S**etting the stage, **E**liciting information, **G**athering information, **U**nderstanding the patient's perspective, and **E**nding the encounter

S-P-I-K-E-S

Setting up, **P**erception, **I**nvitation, **K**nowledge, **E**motions and **S**trategy and summary

ABCDE Model

A - **A**dvance preparation
B - **B**uild a therapeutic environment
C - **C**ommunicate well
D - **D**eals with patient and family reactions
E - **E**ncourage and validate emotions

---

*The GRIEV_ING Model of Death Notification

G — gather

    gather the family; ensure that all members are present.

R—resources

    resources; call for support resources available to assist the family with their grief, i.e., chaplain services, ministers, family and friends.

I—identify

    identify; identify yourself, identify the deceased or injured patient by name, and identify the state of knowledge of the family relative to the events of the day.

E—educate
    educate; briefly educate the family as to the events that have occurred, educate them about the current state of their loved one.

V—verify
    Verify; verify that their family member has died. Be clear! Use the words "dead" or "died."

_—space
    space; give the family personal space and time for an emotional moment; allow the family time to absorb the information.

I—inquire
    inquire; ask if there are any questions, and answer them all.

N—nuts and bolts
    nuts and bolts; inquire about organ donation, funeral services, and personal belongings. Offer the family the opportunity to view the body.

G—give
    give them your card and access information. Offer to answer any questions that may arise later.

The task components to be assessed are likely to vary according to the scenario and task at hand. Whatever the communication skills task is, several of the 27 core objectives listed below are likely to be on the score sheet and you should therefore have them in mind as you conduct the consultation. The examiners expect the candidate to:

1	Establish rapport	15	Find out if patient is willing and able to follow a plan
2	Open discussion	16	Find out what the patient wishes to know
3	Elicit understanding of patient's perception about the illness	17	Use "Ask –Tell-Ask" approach (especially in explaining and teaching)
4	Start with encouraging gestures	18	Give information in plain clear language, at appropriate pace and avoiding use of jargons

5	Show interest and listen attentively	19	Provide aids to enhance understanding
6	Clarify patient's statements	20	Give information layer by layer
7	Show appropriate non-verbal behavior	21	Encourage patient to ask questions
8	Ask about the patient's, fears, emotions and feelings	22	Summarise and check patient's understanding
9	Respond to cues from patient	23	Detail possible treatment options
10	Effectively engage the patient	24	Answer questions truthfully
11	Use open-ended questions appropriately	25	Ensure patient is emotionally stable before ending consultation
12	Use closed questions appropriately	26	Exhibit empathy
13	Demonstrate understanding/knowledge of the issue in question	27	Suggest a follow-up plan and next visit
14	Negotiate and agree with the patient on a plan	28	Appear confident in overall approach to the patient

In the appendices to this chapter, examples of the type of performance expected at some common communication encounters are given. These are only guides and are not meant to be memorised but the general outlines if adopted and used formatively can make your performance at a summative Communication and Ethics station (and during practice) more professional.

4.8. EXAMPLES OF COMMUNICATION SKILLS STATION

A popular communication/ethics task station is delivery of bad news, which we shall use as our first example. The main aspects of the station are the instructions to the candidate, the simulated patient story, and the examiner instructions.

4.8.1. Station X. Delivery of Bad News

Information and Instructions for the Candidate

STATION TITLE: Communication Skills Station
STATION CONSTRUCT OR PURPOSE: This station assesses your ability to break bad news to a patient.

SCENARIO: You are a surgical resident at a University Teaching Hospital. The Medical Team has requested your consultant to review a 50-year-old man, in a medical ward. The patient has had diabetes mellitus for seven years and now presents with a left foot gangrene. After full evaluation, your consultant concludes that the patient needs a below knee amputation to save the patient's life. The doppler test suggests that the femoral and popliteal arteries are adequately patent and therefore good wound healing is expected postoperatively.

YOUR TASK: You are to break the news that his leg is to be amputated, to the patient and deal with any concerns he may have. Do not go into the details of the patient's past history and other areas except as they relate to the intended operation. You are not to seek consent at this stage.

TIME ALLOWED: 5 minutes

Simulated Patient's Profile (This information would not be shown to the candidate)

PERSONAL INFORMATION: You are Mr. Mousa Moudu. Occupation: a surveyor, in own practice. Married, one wife, and three children.

THE PROBLEM.

You are a 50-year-old man, who has had diabetes mellitus for seven years. You are on tablets of Glucophage® 1000 mg twice a day and Amaryl® one tablet once a day for the diabetes. The diabetes appears to be well controlled on these medications. However, six weeks ago you had a minor wound to your left foot. This wound has failed to heal and you have had to be admitted for more treatment. Instead of getting better, the ulcer has become worse. Your physician has to invite a surgeon for advice. After more tests and examinations including a Doppler test, the consultant surgeon has sent his senior registrar (the candidate) to discuss further with you on what the next step should be.

OTHER INFORMATION

The operative death rate in this condition is about one in every 100 but if no operation is performed the patient can expect spreading infection from the foot gangrene causing blood infection and ultimately death. The operation will be followed by fitting of prosthesis and you should be able to go on the prosthesis by eight weeks after the operation. The period of rehabilitation usually takes about six months.

The examiner will rehearse the situation with you before the examination starts.

INFORMATION ABOUT THE CANDIDATE TO BE GIVEN TO THE SIMULATED PATIENT

- Each of the candidate is a senior trainee doctor. They will discuss with you the decision of your doctors about how to manage your foot ulcer which appears to be getting worse.
- You should read the instructions given to the candidate and the examiners to help you better understand what the station is about.
- If requested, please give your name, and other information as in the patient profile provided and as discussed with you.
- Please offer answers only to questions put to you by the candidate and/or ask them those questions you have been told to ask. Please do this consistently and do not volunteer unsolicited information.
- Candidate's task (For information of SP): The duty of the candidate at this examination is to break the bad news, that a right below knee amputation is necessary, to you and deal with any concerns and fears you may have. You have to show concern as previously rehearsed with you.

Information and Instructions for Station Examiner. *This information will not be shown to the candidate, but do take note.*

Your main responsibility as an examiner at this station is to rate the candidate's performance while they interact with the SP as they break the news of amputation to the patient. To be able to do this effectively, you should be familiar with all aspects of this station. Please read all the documents at this station.

Please rate the candidate's performance at executing the task, using the guide provided (Table 4.3) and leaving no components unchecked. In addition to the checklist, *rate globally* the overall performance of the candidate but *independent of* your checklist scores for the candidate at this station. Please enter your global score before the next candidate enters the room.

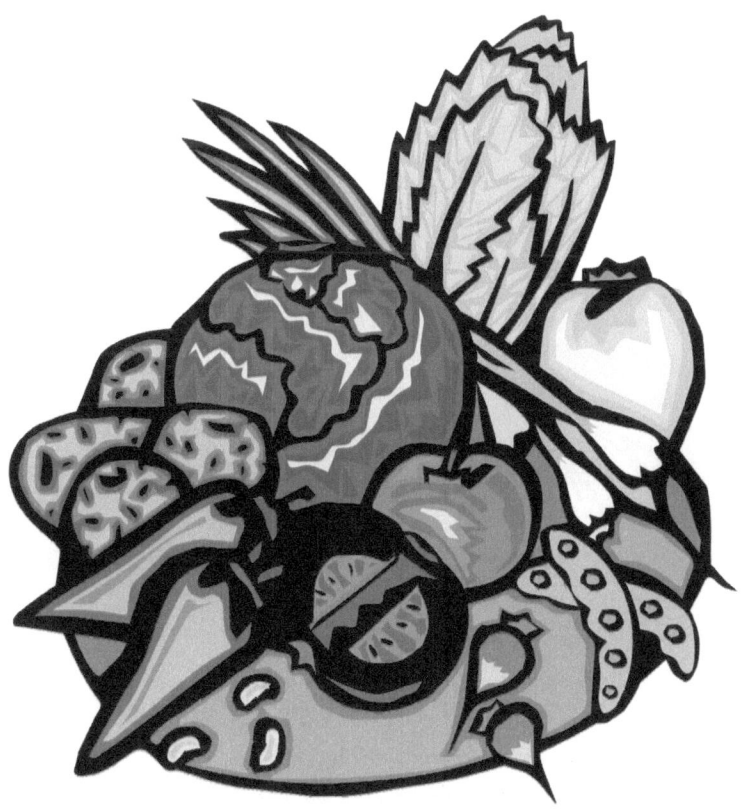

Table 4.3. Assessing Communication Skills at Breaking Bad News (for Postgraduates): *

Task component. *Performance on each item is rated as follows: Very good (5); Good (4); Fair (3); Poorly done (2); Very poor (1); or Not done (0). If item is not applicable indicate NA against it and it will carry no mark.*

OPENS/ESTABLISHES RAPPORT

1. Greets patient. Introduces self. Explains purpose. Asks for patient's name and uses same. Seeks consent,.(5-4-3-2-1-0)
2. **Preparation:** Ensures privacy and no interruptions (switch phones or bleeps off or to silent mode).(5-4-3-2-1-0)
3. Obtains demographics of the patient (3-2-1-0)

BUILDING A THERAPEUTIC ENVIRONMENT/RELATIONSHIP

4. Introduces self to all. Asks for names of others present.(5-4-3-2-1-0)
5. Finds out if patient wants family/ support persons to be present. (5-4-3-2-1-0)
6. Determines what and how much the patient wants to know. (5-4-3-2-1-0)
7. Foreshadows the bad news: Indirectly forewarns that bad news is coming. (3-2-1-0)
8. Uses touch when appropriate. (5-4-3-2-1-0)
9. Schedules follow-up appointments. (5-4-3-2-1-0)

EFFECTIVE COMMUNICATION

10. Asks what the patient already knows before telling and asks what he has told the patient. (Ask-Tell-Ask Approach) (5-4-3-2-1-0)
11. Is frank but compassionate; avoids medical jargon.(5-4-3-2-1-0)
12. Allows for silence and tears, if any; proceeds at the patient's pace. (5-4-3-2-1-0)
13. Has the patient describe their understanding of the news(5-4-3-2-1-0)
14. Allows time to answer questions without interruption;(5-4-3-2-1-0)
15. Encourages patient to ask questions (5-4-3-2-1-0)
16. Writes things down, uses sketches, and provide written information. (5-4-3-2-1-0)
17. Negotiates an agreed follow-up plan(5-4-3-2-1-0)
18. Concludes visit with a summary and follow-up plan.(5-4-3-2-1-0)

Deals with patient and family reactions and concerns

19. Assesses and responds to patient and/or family's emotional reactions.(5-4-3-2-1-0)
20. Deals with coping strategies exhibited by patient.(5-4-3-2-1-0)
21. Shows empathy: verbally and non-verbally (5-4-3-2-1-0)
22. Does not argue with or criticize colleagues' actions.(5-4-3-2-1-0)

COMMUNICATION AND ETHICS

Encouraging and validating emotions

23. Explores what the news means to the patient. (5-4-3-2-1-0)
24. Offers realistic hope according to the patient's goals.(5-4-3-2-1-0)
25. Suggests appropriate use of resources.(5-4-3-2-1-0)
26. Demonstrates knowledge of diabetes and limb amputation (5-4-3-2-1-0)
27. Exhibits knowledge about amputation and subsequent rehabilitation (5-4-3-2-1-0)
28. Tries to ensure that the patient is emotionally fit before bringing the consultation to a close (5-4-3-2-1-0)
29. Provides a clear summary and strategy at the end of the consultation. Provides a proper closure (5-4-3-2-1-0)
30. Answer to Examiner's Question What type of prosthesis would this patient need after BKA?
31. **Global rating** (Excellent (7), Clear pass (6), Borderline pass (5), Borderline fail (4), Clear fail (3), and Abysmal failure (0-2)
32. **Total checklist score for station**

Patterned after the ABCDE Model

The grading of the performance with scores appropriately assigned (Breaking Bad News on Amputation) as applied to undergraduate students might look as follows, that the candidate:

1. Ensures appropriate setting for the type of discussion
2. Confirms patient's name and age
3. Delivers effective introduction and establishes rapport
4. Explores patient's perception and understanding of the situation so far
5. Gives a *warning shot* of what is to come
6. Delivers the bad news
7. Acknowledges and responds to the patients emotional cues
8. Demonstrates empathy both verbally and non-verbally
9. Elicits patient's concerns and worries
10. Effectively uses verbal and nonverbal skills
11. Shows adequate knowledge of diabetes and its complications
12. Shows adequate knowledge of amputation and rehabilitation
13. Gives accurate medical information
14. Uses open and closed questions
15. Gives information in plain language and avoids jargons

16. Gives information in chunks and checks
17. Uses silence effectively
18. Encourages patient to ask questions
19. Maintains rapport throughout with the patient
20. Jointly makes a plan with the patient
21. Summarises the discussion, checking for understanding
22. Provides appropriate and effective closure to the encounter.

Other examples showing core objectives for several themes are shown in appendices 4.1-4.9.

4.9. ADVICE ON HANDLING A COMMUNICATION STATION

4.9.1. General Guides and Hints

1. Communication skill assessment in OSCE is usually with a surrogate patient. Occasionally you may face a real patient; treat both alike as if they were real patients.
2. The thrust of a *Communication and Ethics Skills* station is to test your ability to provide factually correct information, demonstrating professionalism in an effective manner within the emotional context of the clinical setting. Learn the rules.
3. The common types of communication and/or ethics scenarios that you might expect include:
    a. information giving (e.g. please tell this lady about the diagnosis)
    b. delivering bad news (e.g. please inform the patient about the histology report that confirmed the diagnosis of cancer)
    c. Obtaining consent (for a procedure, operation, etc.)
    d. Critical incident (e.g. please talk to the agitated wife of this unconscious patient who was mistakenly given insulin instead of an antibiotic injection).
    e. ethics (e.g. refusal to accept therapy such as having blood transfusion)
    f. confidentiality (disclosing information to a third party)
    g. Education (educate a patient, a relation, or other health professional). Popular ones include use of devices such as peak flow meters and Glucometers.

COMMUNICATION AND ETHICS

4. Read carefully and understand the written *Candidate Instructions* provided about your role, clinical background and the task required. You may make notes from the instructions while waiting for the signal to start.
5. Assessment. As shown in the sample scenarios your performance at this station will be adjudged, depending on the task, on your ability to:
    - select the most appropriate information to communicate
    - provide accurate information
    - explain issues in an appropriate way without medical jargon
    - exhibit empathy
    - respond and adapt to the emotional context of the station and
    - provide a structure to and guide the discussion.
6. Your aim at the station should be to clarify the person's concerns and understanding of the situation, identify and explain clearly the ethical issue or conflict and explore possible solutions.
7. There are many models for the popular communication situations such as educating and teaching; choose and internalise some two or three that will serve your purpose.
8. Always greet the patient warmly, introduce yourself and your role as a candidate. Clarify how they wish to be addressed. Don't forget to also greet the examiners.
9. Make and maintain eye contact throughout the encounter.
10. Use a proper mix of open-ended and closed questions and don't interrupt the patient.
11. If you don't know the answer to a patient's question, be honest and say so.
12. Acknowledge the patient's concerns. Cover FIFE [*Feelings, Ideas, Function, and Expectations*].
13. Actively listen: repeat back, summarize, clarify, paraphrase
14. Take a second to think before you speak.
15. Be aware of your nonverbal cues. In training or practice sessions, you may videotape yourself or ask a partner for feedback.
16. Close the interview with a summary of your findings and the plan of action. Before closing the consultation, always ask the patient "Do you have any other questions?".

17. Lastly and most importantly: practise generously on self, friends and ward or clinic patients before the D-Day

4.9. 2. Active Listening and Empathy

How to Show Someone that You are Actively Listening (*see also s4.9.3*)

1. *Be attentive*:
   - Get rid of all distractions
   - Concentrate on the speaker through natural animation: facial expressions, body language, nodding etc.
   - Appropriately face the speaker
   - Balance comments or talking with silence
   - Maintain natural eye contact
   - Smile when appropriate; avoid frowning

2. *Clarify statements*:
   - Ask for clarification of key words; do not assume
   - Ask for examples
   - Ask for the specific information you need
   - Periodically summarise verbally what you think the speaker has said

3. *Avoid asking "why"*, as this tends to invoke resort to defence mechanisms. Instead recast the question as "what is" or "how is".

How to Show Empathy

- Focus on the patient or speaker and let them know that you are very attentive.
- Allow emotions to be expressed; allow silence and do not interrupt the speaker.
- Get the speaker to come forth with solutions: current and/or in the future.
- Focus on specific needs: "What do you want doctor to do for you?"
- Match the emotional tone set by the patient; let your behaviour indicate that you acknowledge the seriousness or otherwise of the situation.
- Avoid making the patient feel guilty.

4.9. 3. Being an Effective Listener (modified from Haynes)

a. Act like a good listener: Sit relaxed but alert. Make eye contact; make some verbal response...O yes, hmm, is that so? etc.
b. Seek understanding:
   - Hear what is said; listen to what is said; show understanding through empathy or what know.
   - Determine what the speaker means. Clarify words or statements
   - Seek evidence to support what the speaker is saying
   - Identify *what has not been said or deliberately omitted* that might be important.
c. Use time *between* thinking and speaking effectively. Explore concerns. Summarise and play back.
d. Minimise distractions: environmental, endogenous (in the listener) or psychological and distractions from the speaker.
e. Delay judgement until you have heard the speaker out. Do not discountenance the patient's statements.
f. Be patient and allow the speaker time to speak. Know when the patient does not need your help to fill in or provide answers.
g. Pay attention to *how things are said*. Recognise
   - Inflection or emphasis in the patient's voice Speech delivery speed: (fast when excited, angry, or frustrated) or slow (perceived threat, need to think, or lack of interest)
   - Voice pitch (high or low) to gauge stress or being at ease
   - Voice volume- loud when agitated, angry, or excited; and low when depressed, feels threatened, or not wanting others to hear conversation
h. Recognise and observe non-verbal behaviour

4.9. 4. Interpreting Non-verbal behaviour *(NB. Use and interpretation of nonverbal communication would likely vary among cultures. Therefore, some of these may not apply to your own setting. See which ones you agree or do not agree with!)*

1. Leaning forward - involved and interested
2. Leaning back – lack of interest
3. Eye contact:

- Direct eye contact: readiness to engage each other when talking or listening; shows interest or feeling of sincerity and vice versa
- Frequent eye contact indicates confidence and interest.
- Squinting indicates doubt or suspicion.
- Blank stare suggests boredom.

4. Use of hands:
   - Open gestures – open attitude
   - Covering the mouth or tugging at ear – nervousness
   - Touching or rubbing the nose (if not itchy) – suspicion
   - Rubbing the back of the neck – frustration
   - Steepling (bringing the hands so that they touch only at the finger tips) suggests confidence.
   - Touching: hand shake, patting the back etc. – warmth

5. Posture:
   - Tense/rigid or relaxed sitting – stress status
   - Sitting on edge of the chair or leaning forward – cooperation
   - Moving closer – acceptance
   - Turning away from the speaker – suspicion

4.10 CHAPTER FOUR SUMMARY

We may summarise this Chapter on Communication skills and ethics as follows:

- The Communication /ethics station is similar to a history station in structure and will usually have an SP as the patient.
- Effective communication/ethics skills are an integral part of most competencies in clinical practice.
- Communication may be verbal or non-verbal; for every day practice you will need to deploy both skills for you and your patient to engage each other meaningfully.
- The written word as a communication medium is equally important among clinicians and researchers.
- Communication/ethics skills may be assessed as a station standing on its own and/or as part of other competencies like history taking and physical examination skills. You will invariably be examined directly or indirectly on communication /ethics skills. Therefore, prepare well for it.

- The general core communication skills components are: initiating the session, gathering information, building the relationship, explanation and planning, and closing the session. Internalise them.
- More advanced communication skills include breaking bad news, dealing with anger, and dealing with addiction or substance abuse.
- Some forms of Communication are special, such as breaking bad news, educating a patient, and obtaining consent. You will need to develop a system you can use for these special ones in addition to knowing the general rubrics of communication. Adopting and internalising one of the models appropriate for the type of communication will make you perform confidently. Except you are familiar with such models, your performance is likely to be unprofessional and might fetch you marasmic grades unworthy of a good clinician.
- To do well at a communication/ethics station you need to be an effective communicator (i.e. be a good interviewer, use verbal and non-verbal means, be an active and empathetic listener)
- To communicate effectively at OSCE, you need to have practised generously in groups and receive feedback from peers, seniors or even juniors.

4.11. CHAPTER FOUR RECAP EXERCISES

1. What is effective interpersonal communication?
2. List or demonstrate four ways each by which you can pass information to a patient using (a) eye contact and (b) your voice.
3. List the four basic ethical principles.
4. What do the following acronyms representing models for communication stand for?
   (a) ABCDE; (b) SPIKES; and (c) ILS.
5. Which of the models in 4 above will you adopt or adapt for your own use? And why?
6. When educating a patient it is advised that you use the principle of A-T-A. What do these letters standard for?

7. Give one example each of a task at a Communication/ethics Skills Station dealing with (a) Educating a patient; (b) breaking bad news; (c) confidentiality; (d) autonomy; and (e) ethics and the law.
8. List three ways by which you can show empathy.
9. List five characteristics of an effective listener.

4.12. BIBLIOGRAPHY AND RESOURCES: See page 249

4.13. APPENDICES

Appendix 4.1. Refusal To Take Orthodox Medications

Candidate Instructions

SCENARIO: You are the Senior Registrar at the clinic when Mrs Celia Cole, a 64-year-old woman diagnosed with diabetes mellitus five years ago and who has been taking her medications is reported by her son to have abandoned her anti-diabetic tablets and opted instead for a trado-natural medicine practitioner. Her HbA1C is 9% (good control<7%).

YOUR TASK: Please discuss with Mrs Celia Cole her diabetes care.

TIME ALLOWED: 5 minutes

Core objectives on the Examiner's Rating Scale Would Include that the Candidate

CONDUCT OF THE INTERVIEW
1. Makes appropriate introduction, and establishes rapport
2. Explains the purpose of the interview
3. Checks the patient's understanding of diabetes
4. Checks the patient's understanding of the importance of maintaining good glycaemic control
5. Elicits the patient's concerns and worries about the disease
6. Elicits the patient's concerns and worries about the treatment
7. Elicits the patient's beliefs and values with regard to mainstream medicine
8. Explores how Mrs Cole has been taking her medications

9. Gives a clear explanation of diabetes and why it is important to maintain good glycaemic control
10. Discusses lifestyle changes that can help glycaemic control
11. Suggests alternative methods of support or help (e.g. community diabetes nurse, Diabetes Association)
12. Negotiates a joint treatment plan which accommodates Mrs Cole's ideas
13. Makes an appropriate plan for follow-up
14. Summarizes appropriately and periodically

USE OF COMMUNICATION/ETHICS SKILLS
15. Is accurate in information given
16. Avoids using medical jargon
17. Encourages the patient to ask questions
18. Checks for understanding
19. Does not appear patronising or judgemental
20. Is respectful towards the patient's beliefs and values
21. Establishes and maintains rapport with the patient
22. Appropriately and effectively closes the interview

Appendix 4.2. Explanation of an Operative Procedure

Candidate Instructions

SCENARIO: You are the surgical registrar on-call; the ward sister has asked you to speak to Mr Gumo Tashire, who is an elective patient for a laparoscopic cholecystectomy under a general anaesthetic. He is anxious and wishes to discuss the events of the next day with a doctor.

YOUR TASK: Please discuss the pre-operative and postoperative management with him.

TIME ALLOWED: 5 minutes

Core objectives on the Examiner's Rating Scale Would Include that the Candidate

CONDUCT OF THE INTERVIEW
1. Delivers effective introduction and establishes rapport

2. Confirms patient's name and age
3. States the purpose of the interview
4. Elicits patient's own understanding of the operative events
5. Elicits patient's main concerns
6. Explains the need to fast pre-operatively
7. Explains pre-operative medication
8. Explains how the patient will be anaesthetized
9. Offers appropriate explanation of the surgical procedure, including possibility of conversion to open cholecystectomy
10. Explains recovery room procedure (oxygen, blood pressure monitoring etc.)
11. Discusses post-operative analgesia and anti-emetics
12. Explains common post-operative complications

USE OF COMMUNICATION SKILLS
13. Establishes and maintains rapport with the patient
14. Encourages patient to ask questions, and addresses patient's concerns
15. Avoids using medical jargon, and if used explains same
16. Gives accurate medical information
17. Summarizes the discussion appropriately
18. Checks for understanding
19. Appropriately and effectively closes the interview

Appendix 4.3. Explanation of an Investigative Procedure

Candidate Instruction

SCENARIO: You are the Medical Officer assisting the consultant in a clinic. The consultant has just seen a 63-year-old pensioner, Mr John Jidera, who presents with a three-month history of black stools. Mr Jidera has been booked for an upper GI endoscopy.

YOUR TASK: To discuss the procedure with the patient, address any concerns he may have and obtain consent.

TIME ALLOWED: 10 minutes

Core objectives on the Examiner's Rating Scale Would Include that the Candidate

CONDUCT OF THE INTERVIEW
1. Delivers effective introduction and establishes rapport
2. Confirms patient's name and age
3. States the purpose of the interview
4. Elicits patient's own understanding of endoscopy
5. Elicits patient's main concerns
6. Correctly explains bowel preparation to the patient
7. Explains the possibility of intravenous sedation
8. Describes the procedure itself, including the need to take biopsies
9. Explains the post-procedure recovery period
10. Explains to the patient that he will need someone to accompany him home if he receives sedation
11. Explains the risks and benefits of endoscopy procedure
12. Addresses the patient's concern about receiving the result

USE OF COMMUNICATION SKILLS
13. Establishes and maintains rapport with the patient
14. Encourages patient to ask questions and addresses his concerns
15. Avoids using medical jargon
16. Gives accurate medical information
17. Summarizes appropriately
18. Checks for understanding
19. Appropriately and effectively closes the interview

Appendix 4.4. Adherence: Hypertension Management

Candidate Instructions

SCENARIO: You are the medical officer at the MOP asked to see Mrs Justina Jamaru, a known hypertensive patient of several years. There is concern that Mrs Jamaru's blood pressure has been poorly controlled, with the last measurement reading 210/110 mmHg.

YOUR TASK: To explore why Mr Jamaru's blood pressure is poorly controlled, explore any potential complications, and discuss your management plan with her.

TIME ALLOWED 10 minutes

Core objectives on the Examiner's Rating Scale Would Include that the Candidate

1. Gives appropriate introduction and states the purpose of the consultation
2. Confirms patient's name, age and occupation
3. Assesses current status
4. Enquires about his general health
5. Establishes duration of diagnosis of hypertension
6. Enquires about symptoms of complications of hypertension
7. Enquires about symptoms of hypertensive end organ damage
8. Asks to look at self-monitoring results to assess control of hypertension
9. Explores possible reasons for increase in blood pressure
10. Enquires about past medical history
11. Enquires about medication history
12. Enquires about smoking and alcohol history
13. Enquires about diet and level of physical activity
14. Discusses management plan
15. Explains possible reason for increase in blood pressure to the patient
16. Discusses the need for change or continuation of the current treatment as appropriate
17. Explains investigations to be arranged
18. Plans appropriate follow-up
19. Appropriately and effectively closes the interview

NB. This type of assessment can be applied to any station such as diabetes mellitus, asthma, obesity, or any other chronic disease management.

Appendix 4.5. Discharging A Patient On Steroid Therapy

Candidate Instructions

SCENARIO: Mrs Patricia Lopotu is a 51-year-old lady, who was admitted following deterioration of her asthma. She is to be discharged home on bronchodilators and an oral prednisolone dose of 30 mg a day. She is to be seen in three weeks time at the clinic.

YOUR TASK: To discuss the important aspects of steroid therapy with Mrs Lopotu.
TIME ALLOWED: 5 minutes

Core objectives on the Examiner's Rating Scale Would Include that the Candidate that the Candidate:
1. Gives appropriate introduction of self and states the purpose of the interview
2. Confirms patient's name and age
3. Checks patient's understanding of the current situation – admission diagnosis and treatment given in hospital
4. Checks that the patient feels ready to go home
5. Explains the danger of suddenly stopping steroid therapy
6. Explains the risk of intercurrent infection and what to do if she suspects one
7. Explains the possible effect on blood pressure and blood glucose levels
8. Discusses the longterm effect of steroids on bone
9. Discusses the gastrointestinal side effects, and explains the need to cover with a proton pump inhibitor
10. Warns of increased appetite and potential weight gain
11. Warns of skin thinning and risk of bruising
12. Explains to the patient why a steroid bracelet must be worn at all times
13. Ensures that the patient has a steroid card and discusses what it is for
14. Informs patient that she will be followed-up in the Asthma Clinic
15. Addresses the patient's questions and concerns
16. Closes the encounter appropriately

Appendix 4.6. Discharging an Elderly Patient Home

Candidate Instructions

SCENARIO: You are the Registrar working in Ward A2 to which Pa Iputu Ogadu, an 81-year-old man, was admitted with a diagnosis of community acquired pneumonia. He is now fit for discharge.

Your Task: To assess the home situation of Mr Ogadu to help form plans for discharge.
Time allowed: 10 minutes

Core objectives on the Examiner's Rating Scale Would Include that the Candidate

1. Gives appropriate introduction of self and states the purpose of the interview
2. Confirms patient's name and age
3. Establishes patient's understanding of his current medical problems
4. Checks that the patient is aware that discharge is imminent, and explores whether he is happy to go home.
5. Acknowledges patient's concerns and answers any questions

Assesses home situation

6. Asks if the patient lives alone
7. Establishes the type of housing
8. Establishes whether the patient managed independently prior to admission, or whether there was input from social services, a district nurse or anyone else
9. Makes appropriate plan
10. Asks if the patient would like to have input from social services
11. Informs the patient that he will be seen by a physiotherapist and an occupational therapist prior to discharge
12. Gives appropriate medical information
13. States intention to inform patient's Family Physician
14. Makes a sensible plan for follow-up
15. Closes the encounter appropriately

Appendix 4.7. Assessing and Advising on Alcohol

Candidate Instructions

Scenario: Mr James Hassan, a 35-year-old clerical officer, recently lost his job. He appears to be drinking excessively. The wife, worried about the man's behaviour, has convinced him to come and see the doctor, who happens to be you as the Medical Officer in the General Outpatient Clinic.

YOUR TASK: Please take an appropriate history and give advice as necessary and answer the questions put to you by the examiner.

TIME ALLOWED: 10 minutes

Core objectives on the Examiner's Rating Scale Would Include that the Candidate

1. Gives appropriate introduction of self and states reason for the interview
2. Confirms patient's name, age, and occupation/work status
3. Establishes patient's quantity of alcohol intake
4. Establishes pattern of alcohol intake (type, place, time)
5. Deplores the CAGE* questionnaire
6. Enquires about physical symptoms secondary to alcohol misuse
7. Enquires about features of dependence (craving, withdrawal, lessening effect)
8. Establishes social history and enquires about psychosocial impact of alcohol
9. Asks about delusions, hallucinations, and low mood
10. Enquires about past psychiatric history
11. Enquires about past medical history and drug history
12. Gives appropriate advice about safe drinking levels and cutting down

EXAMINER: *WHAT IS YOUR MOST LIKELY DIAGNOSIS?*

13. Answer to question:

EXAMINER: *NAME TWO BIOCHEMICAL AND TWO HAEMATOLOGICAL TESTS THAT MAY SUPPORT YOUR DIAGNOSIS TO BE CARRIED OUT IN THIS PATIENT.*

14. Answers to question:

CLOSURE

15. Closes the encounter appropriately

NB. CAGE Questionnaire:
- Cut down: Have you tried to cut down?

OSCE Skills for Trainees in Medicine

- **A**ngry: Have you felt angry at remarks of others regarding your drinking?
- **G**uilty: Have you felt guilty about how much you drink?
- **E**ye opener: Do you ever drink first thing in the morning?

Appendix 4.8. Teaching A Patient A Technique: PEFR Meter

Candidate Instructions

SCENARIO: Mr. Topade Tayo is a 20-year-old undergraduate who has recently been diagnosed with asthma.

YOUR TASK: Explain to Topade how to use a peak expiratory flow rate (PEFR) meter in the management of his asthma.

TIME ALLOWED: 5 minutes

Core objectives on the Examiner's Rating Scale Would Include that the Candidate

1. Establishes rapport; obtains patient's demographics
2. Establishes the purpose of the consultation
3. Checks patient's understanding of asthma
3. Explains importance of PEFR meter and how it works
5. Explains when PEFR meter is to be used
4. Identifies the components of the instruments
5. Establishes what the patient already knows about PEFR meter
6. Demonstrates the procedure silently while the patient watches
7. Breaks the procedure into steps and explains each step
8. Explains again and demonstrates each step as follows:
    8a. Explains and demonstrates how to attach a clean mouthpiece
    8b. Slides the marker down to the bottom of the numbered scale
    8c. Stands or sits up straight
    8d. Holds the meter horizontal
    8e. Takes as deep a breath as possible
    8f. Seals lips around mouthpiece
    8g. Exhales as hard as possible into the meter
    8h. Reads and records the meter reading
9. [Now] Asks the patient to *explain the procedure*
10. Asks the patient to *demonstrate the procedure*

COMMUNICATION AND ETHICS

11. [Offers] to go over the above steps several times until the patient and doctor are satisfied
12. Explains need to repeat procedure at least three times
13. Checks reading against peak flow chart or previous readings
14. Discusses common problems and how to fix them
15. Tests the patient's understanding again
16. Invites questions and comments
17. Summarises the session
18. Closes the encounter appropriately

Appendix 4.9. Counselling a Patient and Obtaining Consent

Instructions to the Candidate

SCENARIO: Mr Peter Kotu is a 25-year-old student. He has come to donate blood because his sister is to have an operation that will require being transfused with blood. To be eligible for blood donation, testing for Hepatitis B virus among others is required.

YOUR TASK: Counsel Mr Palotu before he is tested and obtain his consent.

TIME ALLOWED: 5 minutes

Core objectives on the Examiner's Rating Scale Would Include that the Candidate

1. Establishes rapport
2. Explains purpose of the meeting
3. Assures confidentiality
4. Assesses risk
5. Discusses the disease (Hepatitis B virus infection)
6. Explains the test
7. Discusses the legal, financial, and social implications of test
8. Discusses the consequences of positive and negative Hepatitis B testing
9. Requests for consent
10. Advises about behaviour pending test result (if applicable)
11. Summarises the encounter
12. Provides good closure

Appendix 4. 10. Generic Objectives for Assessment of "Explaining a Diagnosis, an Investigation and/or Treatment" *(Adequate, 2; Inadequate, 1; and Not done, 0)*

The candidate:

1.	Assumes professional sitting position	(S-BL-UNS-NP)
2.	Establishes rapport	(S-BL-UNS-NP)
3.	Explains task or purpose of meeting	(S-BL-UNS-NP)
4.	Obtains consent to proceed	(S-BL-UNS-NP)
5.	Determines what the patient already knows	(S-BL-UNS-NP)
6.	Offers clear, structured, step-by-step explanation	(S-BL-UNS-NP)
7.	Uses proper language, avoids jargons	(S-BL-UNS-NP)
8.	Asks periodically for patient's understanding by repeating the information back to candidate	(S-BL-UNS-NP)
9	Seeks and addresses patient's concerns and expectations	(S-BL-UNS-NP)
10.	Addresses task-specific content items	(S-BL-UNS-NP)
11.	Clarifies and summarises discussion	(S-BL-UNS-NP)
12.	Provides appropriate closure	(S-BL-UNS-NP)
13	Exhibits respect and courtesy throughout encounter	(S-BL-UNS-NP)

(S, satisfactory, B; borderline; UNS, unsatisfactory; NP, not performed)

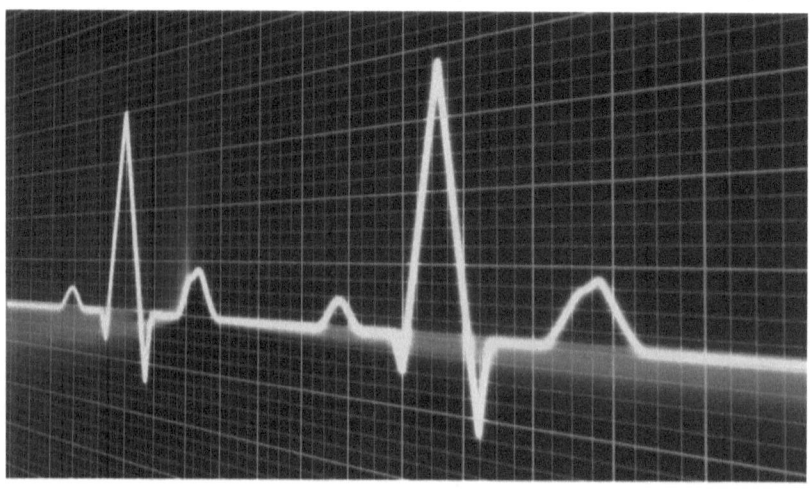

5

Physical Examination Skills Station

5.1. Physical Examination in Trainee Assessment

5.2. Types of Physical Examination Station

5.3. Essentials at a Physical Examination Skills Station

5.4. What Physical Examination Station is Testing

5.5. Hints on Physical Examination Skills

5.6. Assessing Physical Examination Skills

5.7. An Example of Physical Examination Skills Station

5.8. Chapter Five Summary

5.9. Chapter Five Recap Exercises

5.10. Bibliography and Resources

5.11 Appendices

5.1. PHYSICAL EXAMINATION IN TRAINEE ASSESSMENT

A physical examination (PE) station (Fig 5.1) is a constant feature of most OSCEs for both undergraduate and postgraduate medical trainees. Here is the station where you have the opportunity to demonstrate what you can do at the bedside under direct observation. Physical examination stations are useful for assessment at all phases of medical training. The objective of assessment at this station can range from demonstration of physical signs or showing how it should be done to eliciting abilities, situating the findings in context and planning management.

There are differences between routine physical examination and PE as applied to OSCE. Given the limited time available in OSCE, it is not expected to examine from head to toe even if some appear to contribute little to resolving the problem at hand. In OSCE, the emphasis is on a *focussed and relevant clinical examination* with stress on relevant data gathering in the context of a given problem. Physical examination requires the exhibition of the candidate's medical knowledge concerning the specific patient problem and the physical manifestations of a disorder. The examiners are looking for a fluid and competent performance and (if required or asked) a clear and confident presentation of the findings, differential diagnoses, and management plan. Performing a PE on a patient when other people are present may appear difficult but with practice one can overcome the inhibition. Running a commentary for people to hear helps partly to overcome this hurdle.

5.2. PURPOSE AND TYPES OF PHYSICAL EXAMINATION STATION

Purpose of Physical Examination Skills Station

Physical examination stations can be used to assess student performance *formatively and summatively*. The PE station is useful for assessing several clinical skills at the *shows how* level of Miller's pyramid of competencies. A PE skills station can be designed to assess one or more competencies at an encounter but generally a PE station purpose tends to be limited to one primary task and one or two secondary tasks. In complexity, PE stations may vary from the inspection level to demonstration of more difficult manoeuvres.

PHYSICAL EXAMINATION STATION

There can be several types of physical examination encounters in an OSCE. The task is defined by the purpose of the particular station. The common skills that are often examined at PE stations include:
- Ability to formulate a management plan
- Ability to present the findings
- Communication skills as part of the physical examination
- Conducting the physical examination using appropriate aids
- Correctly interpreting physical examination findings
- Demonstrating respect/concern for the patient and their safety, comfort, and modesty.
- Eliciting relevant and specific abnormalities
- Performance of an appropriate, focussed, and systematic examination
- Reducing transmission of infection at least before and at the end of the examination

The following are the usual types of Physical Examination Skills Stations:
- Demonstration of a procedure or technique e.g. measurement of JVP
- Examination of a whole system: e.g. cardiovascular, gastrointestinal
- Examination of an aspect of a system e.g. motor system, abdomen, a mass
- General physical examination
- Probe or couplet station, following another station
- Regional examination e.g. face, neck, abdomen, foot
- Subthemes of general examination e.g. lymph nodes, nutritional status

A physical examination station may be linked to a follow-up station using written questions, oral presentation, interpretation of physical signs etc.

5.3. ESSENTIALS AT A PHYSICAL EXAM STATION

At the physical examination skills (PES) station you will meet staff / examiners, a number of information items and physical examination aids.

Staff at a Physical Examination Station

Examination-related persons at the **physical examination station** include the patient, examiners, and assistants.

PATIENTS AT PHYSICAL EXAMINATION STATION

The OSCE physical examination patient may be a real or simulated one. Simulated patients at PES station are made to feign physical signs. Among the physical signs that can be mimicked are the following:

- Gait changes
- Hearing loss
- Hyperaesthesia
- Lid lag
- Memory changes
- Pleuritic chest
- Sensory loss (touch)
- Tenderness
- Tremors
- Visual loss

OSCE EXAMINERS AND ASSISTANTS

Examiners at a PES station are usually persons with knowledge of the process and content of a physical examination, i.e. clinicians. However, others including SPs may be trained to do the rating as well using a checklist. You should relate to any examiner as you would to your teacher.

Information Items at Physical Examination Station

The following body of written information or some modification of it is likely to be present at the PE station:

a. Station Title and Station Number
b. Station Construct or Purpose
c. Candidate Instructions including the Patient Scenario/Setting
d. Patient instructions (Not available to candidate)
e. Examiner instructions (Not available to candidate)
f. Analytical checklist or rating scale (not available to candidate)
g. Evaluation or Feedback forms (usually one for the whole OSCE).

The *Station Title* gives the broad competency domain the station is to assess, e.g. physical examination skills. *Station Construct* describes the purpose of the station: e.g. to assess the ability of the candidate to conduct a neurological examination on a patient. The item that directly concerns the candidate most is *the Candidate Instruction* including the patient scenario and setting.

Briefing Instructions for the Candidate

The *Candidate Instructions* would consist of the patient scenario/setting including what designation is assigned to the candidate. The instruction is likely to be succinctly set out in three to four sentences, stating clearly

what the problem is and what task you are to perform or undertake and the time available as follows:
- Station number: as on the OSCE circuit
- Station title: Physical Examination
- Time allowed: 5/10/15 minutes
- Station Construct: "This station tests your ability to conduct an abdominal examination on a patient who complains of abdominal pain".

A sample instruction to the candidate at a PES Station might look like the following:

CLINICAL SCENARIO: You are the junior resident on duty at the ED of a teaching hospital when Mr Sakpan presents to the facility late in the night complaining of abdominal pain. He admits to taking a number of drugs for several years to treat the pain but the pain became worse recently.

Your Task: Do a focussed abdominal examination of the patient; tell the examiners what you are doing and why. The examiners besides scoring your performance will ask you a few questions before you leave the station. If you need any help, please ask the examiner.

TIME ALLOWED: You have FIVE minutes at this station.

Information for the Patient at a Physical Examination Station

The instructions to the patient at an OSCE physical examination station are often precise and succinct. Most (if any) of the interaction with the candidate will require the patient answering just a few questions or obeying simple instructions.

Only body parts to be examined need be exposed at a given time. The patient must have been briefed on how to react if you are doing otherwise. You must ensure, in all these, *patient's modesty and comfort*. Ensure appropriate draping, limiting exposure to just the areas under focus at a given time; avoid inflicting pain on the patient (if you must have their co-operation). Do not expect any prompting from either the patient or the station examiner, but they may halt you if you pose a threat to patient safety, comfort, or modesty. That can cost you the station.

OSCE Skills for Trainees in Medicine

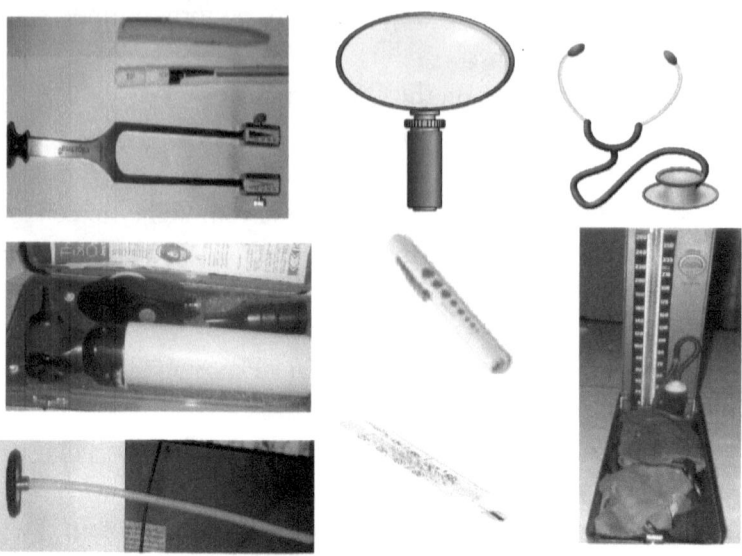

Figure 5.1. Physical Examination Diagnostics. *A variety of instruments and devices may be made available to assist you at the physical examination station. It is up to you to decide which one to use.*

Materials and Diagnostics at a Physical Examination Station

At the PES station you will expect to find standard OSCE station materials including chairs, couch or beds, and equipment/devices for physical examination (See Figure 5.1.). The organisers will usually provide more materials than what you need for the examination such as:

SUPPLIES AND MATERIALS
- Lubricating jelly
- Materials for washing hands
- Mydriatic solution
- Paper towels
- Rectal gloves
- Tape measure
- Tissues
- Tongue depressors
- Vials of coffee and cinnamon

EQUIPMENT AND DEVICES
- Flashlight
- Monofilament
- Neurotips
- Oto-ophthalmoscope
- Pocket eye chart
- Reflex hammers
- Sphygmomanometer
- Stethoscope
- Thermometer
- Tuning fork (128 /256/512Hz)

It will be up to you to decide which equipment you need to use. If you are allowed to use your own equipment such as a stethoscope and an ophthalmoscope, it is advisable then that you use them as you would have become very familiar with their use.

5.4. OBJECTIVE OF THE PHYSICAL EXAMINATION STATION

Examiners' Expectations

The examiners will observe and grade your interaction with the patient and may ask you a few questions if that is built into the checklist. The examiners expect you among others to:

- Introduce yourself to the patient
- Tell the patient what you are going to do; and seek their permission.
- Drape the patient appropriately, exposing areas only as and if needed.
- Ask the patient to remove clothing, but not to remove their clothing for them unless required.
- Help the patient on and off the examination table.
- Be systematic, organized, and try not to have the patient constantly changing positions for your examination
- If required be fluent, confident, and succinct in presentation of your findings and offer sensible differential diagnoses.

OSCE Skills for Trainees in Medicine

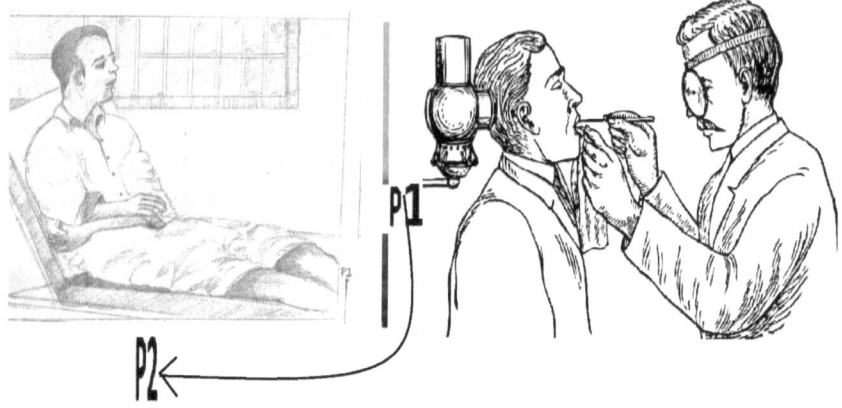

Figure 5.2. Positioning of a Clinician when Performing a Physical Examination. *It is traditional to start physical examination from the foot of the bed for general inspection (P1 on left panel). Thereafter move to the right side of the patient to carry out further physical assessment (P2 on left panel). Always examine from the right side of the patient, even if you are a left-handed person. However this positioning is not immutable, patients when thought appropriate may be examined sitting down, standing (right panel) or in the arms of parents.*

Positioning the Patient and Yourself

For most PEs, the patient is supine while you stand at their right hand side (Fig 5.1). But this positioning is not invariable as the optimum positioning will depend on what you are examining and the comfort of the patient. Table 5.1 shows some of the common positions during physical examination.

Table 5.1. Positioning Doctor and Patient for a Physical Examination

Nature of activity	Patient	Examiner	Remarks
Hand washing		In front of patient	Before and after;
Vital signs, general inspection	Sitting or reclining	Stand before patient or at bedside	patient to be supine inspect from foot of bed
Head and neck	Sitting	Stand before patient	May be part of general examination
Anterior torso	Sitting	Stand before patient initially	(Inspection± palpation)
Posterior torso	Sitting	At patient's side	(Inspection± palpation)
Abdomen	Supine	At patient's right side	Start from end of bed, then before the patient
Anterior Chest	At 45^0	At patient's right side	Start from end of bed, then move to the side
Posterior chest	Sitting (in bed)	At patient's right side	
Male genitalia	Standing	Before the patient	
Gait, station, coordination (GALS)	Variable positions	Variable positions	Check on GALS* (for musculoskeletal)
Female genitalia	Reclining on examining table, feet in stirrups	Sit on stool or stand	Patient, draped, knees flexed, legs adducted
Heart	Lying at 45^0	Stand to the right	
Thyroid	Sitting	Stand in front, by the side and behind	Ask for water if not provided
Fundi	Sitting	Stand in front	Bring your own ophthalmoscope

*GALS: Gait, Arms, Legs, and Spine

5.5. HINTS ON PHYSICAL EXAMINATION SKILLS

Preparation ahead of the OSCE
1. To do well at the PES station, you must have prepared well for the exercise, i.e. practised frequently and seriously.
2. Practise on fellow trainees and patients (under supervision).
3. Make a list of the common PES tasks and organise and master how these would be handled if you are asked to do any (See Appendix 5.4).
4. Clip your fingernails before the examination.
5. Wear appropriate clothing and maintain a professional appearance.
6. Avoid perfumes/cologne except if you have body odour; even then do not use strong perfumes.
7. Do not put on hand jewellery during the OSCE session especially at PE stations.
8. Most if not all instruments and materials required for a particular station will be provided but you may want to use your own stethoscope. Bring a stethoscope with separate bell and diaphragm heads.

At the Physical Examination Skills Station
9. Read the "instructions to the candidate" very carefully. Ascertain if you may make notes on completing the examination.
10. Introduce yourself to the patient; seek permission.
11. Be polite, considerate, and respectful.
12. Acknowledge the patient's concerns.
13. Wash your hands with soap or use hand sanitizers in front of the patient before starting (and after) the physical examination.
14. Position the patient and yourself properly.
15. Always use patient gowns and drapes appropriately to maintain patient modesty and comfort.
16. Never examine through the patient's gown; place stethoscope directly on the patient's skin not over clothing.
17. *Talk before you touch*. Tell the patient when you are ready to begin the physical examination and what you are going to do at every stage.

18. Do a focused physical examination based on the scenario and task before you.
19. Describe the manoeuvres either before or as you perform them to the examiner (or do as the instructions say).
20. Try and use all the allotted time. Use any extra time to mentally review your performance; you may be able to add some important points. Feel free to go back (with the patient's permission) and perform any examination aspect that you might have omitted.
21. Be systematic and organized; try not to have the patient constantly changing positions for your examination.
22. If you believe a sensitive or stressful examination (such as a rectal, pelvic/genital, or female breast examination) is indicated, tell the examiner. The examiners are given instructions on how to deal with such situations. You will not be expected to perform such procedures in live persons during the OSCE but you should know them as alternatives may be provided. You will be awarded some marks for just expressing the intention to do so!
23. If you ask a patient to lie back on the examination table, pull the leg rest out, then help the patient sit back up and return the leg rest. Help the patient on and off the examination table.
24. Close the encounter appropriately including summarising your findings to the patient and thanking them for their cooperation.

Miscellaneous Tips on Physical Examination in OSCE

1. Organisating the Physical Examination

AT INITIATION OF THE PHYSICAL EXAMINATION:
Deploy a mnemonic such as **WIPER** to help you:

W - *Wash* your hands.

I - *Introduce* yourself to the patient. Greet the patient (title and surname).

P – *Permission*: Explain what you would like to do. Obtain consent for the examination.

Pain: Ask the patient if they are in *any pain* and to tell you if they experience any during the examination.

E - *Expose* the necessary parts of the patient. Ideally the patient should be undressed from the waist up taking care to ensure the patient is not cold or unnecessarily embarrassed.

R - *Reposition* the patient as appropriate for the target of examination. (See Table 5.1)

2. Performing the specified task

a. Use a focussed approach to the examination.
b. Follow the usual sequence of examination, (Inspection, Palpation, Percussion, and Auscultation) modified as appropriate.
c. Explain to the patient what you are about to do at each stage without using jargon.
d. Avoid causing pain or embarrassment to the patient. Again ask the patient if they have any pain, and examine gently to start with.
e. Look at the patient's face and ask them to let you know if they feel any pain especially when feeling for tenderness.

3. Closing the Physical Examination Encounter

a. Decide/determine if you need to examine any system in more detail e.g. a patient with proptosis.
b. If there is time, re-examine any aspect that you are unsure about.
c. Tell the patient when you have completed your examination.
d. Tell the patient what you found and what next to follow.
e. Express your appreciation to them and help reposition/dress them if needed.
f. Wash your hands once more.

4. Preparing to Present Findings and/or to Face the Examiners

a. Summarise your findings in a few lines; use the SOAP approach.
b. List a few differential diagnoses for the findings
c. Make a problem list (**A**ssessment component of SOAP)
d. Make a management plan (P arm of SOAP) consisting of
   i. Tests required to confirm or establish the diagnosis /aetiology
   ii. Treatment that should be given to the patient.
   iii. Patient education
   iv. Referrals/consultations, if any indicated

5. Sundry Tips
   a. For each body system or region make a potential OSCE station list.
   b. Memorise and rehearse the normal physical examination sequence expected for each system or region.
   c. Practise the physical examination of each system in the expected time allowed.
   d. Practise explaining what you are doing, what you are feeling/listening for and thinking as you perform the physical examination.
   e. Before presentation, do rehearse in your mind what abnormal findings might mean in terms of differential diagnoses and how to present the findings coherently *(vide supra)*

5.6. ASSESSMENT OF PHYSICAL EXAMINATION SKILLS

Assessing the candidate's performance at the PES station is usually done by one or two trainers but other health professionals may be used and in some centres a trained simulated patient may also do the rating. In formative assessment, scoring may also be done by your peers. Scoring is done using *checklists, rating scales, global rating*, or some combination of these.

Scoresheets may contain structured questions with clear expected answers that the examiner may ask you, in the last few moments of the encounter. Such questions are often in the following form: summarise your findings; what is your most likely diagnosis; or how will you manage this patient? At the end of your examination ask yourself these questions before facing the examiners.

Assessment Domains of Physical Examination Skills

We mentioned earlier that the PE procedure at the OSCE station necessarily differs from the routine traditional method of examination. Some aspects of the examination must, however, follow the traditional pattern e.g. inspection before palpation. Examination should be conducted in such a way as to reduce stress to the patient and must, therefore, be focussed. Thus all aspects of the anterior or posterior chest should be examined once rather than dealing with CVS and coming back to examine the respiratory system. The OSCE physical examination structure consists essentially of:

- the general/introductory/communication/ part,
- the specific task content components and
- ending the encounter section.

When required, the PE station may be followed by a presentation at the same station or at the next (couplet) station. Presentation of findings should be logically done as to make sense; be prepared to synthesise your findings in a short discussion that might follow.

The physical examination process, for the purpose of assessment or scoring, is usually broken down into a number of objectives such as:
- Communication: establishing rapport (at start and throughout the process)
- Making the patient at ease all throughout
- Explaining the purpose of the encounter and seeking consent
- Making the patient comfortable in required position
- Hand washing or cleaning
- Going through the traditional rhythm of IPPA
- Synthesising of findings to formulate a problem list and to make a diagnosis
- Explaining the findings and their implications to the patient.
- Properly and politely ending the examination session

Each of these objectives would be scored. As you go through the routine of the PE, be thinking of these aspects on which your assessment is likely to be based.

Assessment Approach to Physical Examination Skills

As is usual for all OSCE assessments, the task is broken down into easily discernible and assessable components or objectives. Task components may be differentially weighted (based on the degree of perceived importance of the component to the execution of the task). Among what the examiners are generally expecting of you at a PE skills station and for which marks would be awarded (or lost) are the following:

GENERAL/INTRODUCTORY/COMMUNICATION ASPECTS
- Establishing initial rapport: greets patient, introduces self and explains the purpose.

- Asks for patient's name, and seeks consent
- Explaining to the patient what examination will be carried out
- Washing hands before beginning physical examination
- Draping the patient appropriately during each segment of the PE

PERFORMANCE ON COMPONENTS OF THE STATION-SPECIFIC TASK E.G.
- Proper positioning of patient
- Sequentially performing tasks

GENERAL TECHNICAL ASPECTS OF THE PERFORMANCE
- Organization of the PE (if smooth, appropriate, systematic and focused)
- Process of eliciting relevant and specific findings
- Ability to distinguish normal from abnormal findings
- Attention to patient's physical comfort and dignity/modesty
- Relationship to the patient

PROPER CLOSURE
- Summarising and clarifying the findings to the patient
- Describing what next to follow
- Acknowledging patient
- Closing encounter politely

INTERACTION /DISCUSSION (AT THE SAME OR THE FOLLOWING STATION)
- (If required) ability to present findings coherently
- Ability to interpret physical signs correctly
- Ability to formulate differential diagnoses, and/or problem list
- Ability to select relevant cost effective investigations in an appropriate sequence
- Ability to choose appropriate management options

While the standard traditional sequence of inspection from a defined position, palpation, percussion, auscultation and special manoeuvres may be appropriate for the chest, in the abdomen the sequence is best as *inspection from appropriate position, auscultation, palpation, percussion,* and special manoeuvres. Percussion may not carry much importance in

OSCE Skills for Trainees in Medicine

examination of some organs e.g. the heart, skin or joints. So appropriately adapt the examination.

The level of achievement of each of the objectives may be scored in a number of ways such as excellent (5 marks); good (4 marks); fair (3 marks); poor (2 marks); very poor, (1 mark); and not performed (0 mark).

5.7. AN EXAMPLE OF A PHYSICAL EXAMINATION SKILLS STATION

To illustrate the general principles of assessing PES station, we shall take a patient presenting with abdominal pain. The information available to the candidate will include:

General Station Elements *and* Instruction to the Candidate
General Station Elements
a. Station number: IX
b. Station title: Physical Examination Station
c. Station construct: The purpose of this station is to test the candidate's ability to complete a focused abdominal examination in a patient who presents with abdominal pain.
d. Time allowed: 5 minutes

Information and Instructions for the Candidate
STATION NUMBER: IX
STATION TITLE: Physical Examination
TIME ALLOWED: 5 minutes
STATION CONSTRUCT: This station tests your ability to conduct an abdominal examination on a patient who complains of abdominal pain.
CLINICAL SCENARIO: You are a junior resident on duty at the ED of a teaching hospital. Mr Akpani presents to you late in the night complaining of abdominal pain.

YOUR TASK:
i. Do a focussed abdominal examination of the patient
ii. Explain what you are doing to the patient as you go and say to the hearing of the examiners what you are doing and why.

iii. Summarise your findings for the patient at the end of the examination.
iv. Give the patient some advice about your findings.
v. Answer any questions the examiners may ask you about the patient and/or make notes of your findings for the next station

Note that:
- A full history is NOT required, but questions relevant to the proposed examination may be asked.
- The examiners besides scoring your performance will ask you a few question when you have completed your examination.
- If you need any help or particular material or equipment, ask the examiner.
- **Scoring Information**: (This information is usually part of the pre-OSCE briefing to all candidates and is not likely to be shown at the station.)
- *Analytical Rating Scale or Checklist.* On each task component on the score sheet, you will be scored as follows: *Very good, Good, Fair, Poor, Very poor or not performed* for execution of any component of the station task.
- *Global Rating.* Besides semi-quantitatively rating your performance at each task component, you will be rated globally as *excellent pass; Good pass; Borderline pass; Borderline fail; Clear fail;* or *Abysmal fail*. Global rating is done without reference to your total checklist scores for this purpose.

Information for the Patient at Physical Examination Station IX

The following information is for the attention of the standardised patient.

"You are Mr Ado Akpani, a 45-year-old police officer. You have had abdominal pain for over five years. You take several drugs for this pain; these drugs have generally been helpful but in the last three months the pain has become worse and was so severe last night you had to be brought into ED. No tests have yet been done. You have had some injection and the pain is now less. As part of the initial assessment the doctor is going to examine your abdomen to see if any additional information about the abdominal pain can be obtained.

OSCE Skills for Trainees in Medicine

Table 5.2. Assessment of Physical Examination of the Abdomen

Task component item/Activity	Performance Score				
Note that applicability of item would vary with the characteristics of the patient being used.	VG	Good	Fair	Poor	VP/ND
1. **Opens/establishes rapport.** Greets patient, introduces self, Asks for and uses patient's name; Explains purpose of encounter and seeks consent	5	4	3	2	0
General/Communications skills					
2. Washes hands before and after examining the patient or uses alcohol wipes	3	2	1	1	0
3. **Ensures optimal conditions:** lighting; quiet environment, etc.	5	4	3	2	0
4. **Ensures patient modesty and comfort.** Asks for a chaperon if of opposite sex to be present. Drapes and undrapes patient properly	5	4	3	2	0
5. Explains examination manoeuvres clearly, transits smoothly; allows patient to accommodate ___	5	4	3	2	0
EXAMINATION TECHNIQUES					
6. **Appropriate positioning** of patient and self (supine with one pillow). Begins assessment at patient's right.	3	2	2	1	0
7. **Sequence:** Follows the abdominal examination sequence of: Inspection, Auscultation, Percussion, and Palpation. Systematically examines all abdominal regions.	5	4	3	2	0
8. **Inspection.** Systematically inspects and comments on: Patient's abdominal symmetry, skin, masses and contour.	5	4	3	2	0
AUSCULTATION. USES THE DIAPHRAGM OF THE STETHOSCOPE AND AUSCULTATES FOR AND COMMENTS ON:					
9. Bowel sounds, abdominal aorta, renal artery, and femoral artery bruits	5	4	3	2	0
PERCUSSES THE ABDOMEN FOR AND COMMENTS ON:					
10. Tone in all quadrants, gastric air bubble, suprapubic dullness	5	4	3	2	0
11. Liver span	5	4	3	2	0
12. Splenic dullness	5	4	3	2	0
PALPATION					
13. Asks for any areas of tenderness	5	4	3	2	0
14. General technique (position of candidate's hand, starting point)	5	4	3	2	0
15. Does light and deep palpation	5	4	3	2	0
16. Does bimanual palpation and balloting of both kidneys	5	4	3	2	0
17. Palpates for splenic enlargement	5	4	3	2	0

PHYSICAL EXAMINATION STATION

18	Palpates for aortic and femoral arteries and para-aortic glands	5	4	3	2	0
19	Palpates for pelvic masses (urinary bladder, uterus etc.) and palpates both groins	5	4	3	2	0
	SPECIAL TESTS (MAY ONLY BE DONE IF INDICATED)					
20	Inspects abdominal muscles as patient raises head to detect: masses, hernia, separation of muscles, veins	5	4	3	2	0
21	Tests for fluid wave and/or shifting dullness	5	4	3	2	0
22	Employs methods to relax abdomen: open mouth breathing, knees flexed	5	4	3	2	0
23	Tests for Murphy sign and tests for right costovertebral angles for kidney tenderness	5	4	3	2	0
24	Palpates for tenderness over gallbladder region	5	4	3	2	0
25	Tests for asterixis	5	4	3	2	0
26	Requests to examine external genitalia	3	3	2	1	0
27	Seeks permission to do a digital rectal examination	5	4	3	2	0
28	Does a focussed general examination: hands, face, neck for lymph nodes and legs/feet	5	4	3	2	0
29	Organization of Physical Examination	5	4	3	2	0
30	Relationship to the Patient	5	4	3	2	0
31	Summary, Strategy, and closure	8	5	3	2	0
32	What is the most likely diagnosis?	5	4	3	2	1
33	GLOBAL RATING: Excellent; Good; Borderline pass; Borderline fail; Clear fail; Abysmal fail					
34	Maximum analytical score for station					
35	Candidate's score					
General Comments on candidate (non-scoring) or station						
Name of Examiner			Signature of Examiner			Date

VG, very good; VP, very poor; ND, not done.

The trainee will not be required to obtain a full history from you, but your answers to specific questions, if asked, may include:
- Your name, age, occupation and complaint
- You do not suffer from any other pain
- The pain is made worse by hunger but relieved by food or antacid
- Your general health is good.

Seek clarification from the candidate at any stage if anything said or done seems unclear. If they do not otherwise do so, you may ask them why they are doing a particular examination, or what they are looking for. Also feel free to indicate if any part of the examination is uncomfortable or painful. You should read the instructions to the candidate and the marksheet before the examination starts".

Information and Instructions for Station Examiner

(This information is *not available* to the candidate at the OSCE station).
- Please read all the other briefings and information items at this station.
- Do not prompt any of the candidates except as previously agreed to by all.
- Score the performance of the candidate using the marksheet provided (Table 5.2).
- Please do the global rating before totalling your analytical scores; the latter might best be done at the end of the circuit. Enter component and global rating scores independently.
- You should enter you global score before the next candidate enters the room

Note that not all the signs shown in Table 5.2 would be present depending on the findings; one finding may inform the search for another. The presence of jaundice calls for eliciting asterixis while absence of dullness in the flanks renders demonstrating shifting dullness redundant.

5.8. CHAPTER FIVE SUMMARY

- The physical examination skills (PES) station is a constant feature of most OSCE exercises.
- Patients at PES station may be simulated or real and may not have abnormal physical signs. Emphasis may be on the process of eliciting physical signs.
- The PES station can be used to assess medical knowledge, communication skills, approach to physical examination, interpretation of the findings and how these should inform management plan.
- At the PES station the examiners expect you to be able to identify and interpret physical signs, to demonstrate professionalism, respect for patient including their safety, comfort, and modesty.
- When challenged you should be able to present the findings and formulate a management plan.

- The key to doing well at a PES encounter is frequent practice on the common areas or systems for examination. Develop and use a system that works best for you and yet formal.
- Read also the relevant section in the Chapter 10 on PACES.
- Be conversant with what brings good or poor scores (Appendix 5)

5.9. CHAPTER FIVE RECAP EXERCISES

1. What is the major difference between routine physical examination (PE) and PE in an OSCE setting?
2. List four main aspects for which you are likely to be scored at a physical examination skills (PES) station.
3. Hand washing is an important skill for PES station. When and how should this be done?
4. If told to examine the abdomen in a woman, how would you ensure her modesty?
5. What is your own system for presenting your findings at a PES station?
6. In terms of sequence, how is examination of the abdomen different from examination of the chest?

5.10. BIBLIOGRPHY AND RESOURCES see page 249

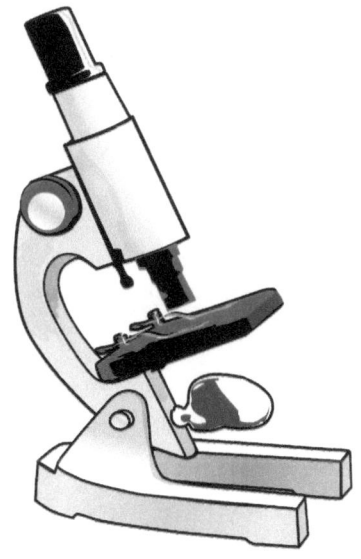

5.11. APPENDICES

Appendix 5.1. Template for Scoring Performance at a Physical Examination Station

Example of a Grading System: Very good, 5; Good, 4; Average, 3; Poor, 2; Very poor, 1; Not performed, 0. You can modify this for your rehearsal.

GENERAL ASPECTS OF PHYSICAL EXAMINATION
1. Opens/establishes rapport. Greets patient. Introduces self. Asks for patient's name. Uses patient's name; Explains purpose of encounter and seeks consent
2. Establishes rapport throughout the process and makes the patient at ease, acknowledges distress, respects modesty
3. Obtains patient's demographics
4. Makes patient comfortable and in required position
5. Washes hands (before and after physical examination)
6. Observes patient's general appearance and behaviour; comments on signs of illness/distress
7. Draping and disrobing: Informs and seeks patient's permission and co-operation
8. Explains examination manoeuvres clearly, transits smoothly; allows patient to accommodate.
9. Goes through the traditional rhythm of physical examination in a focussed and systematic manner

DOES A FOCUSSED EXAMINATION OF THE ORGAN, SYSTEM OR REGION REQUIRED AS FOLLOWS AND/OR AS APPROPRIATE:
10. Inspection
11. Palpation
12. Percussion
13. Auscultation
14. Special procedures
15. Does a focussed general examination related to task
16. Demonstrates expertise in the organization of physical examination of the organ/system/ region

CLOSURE

17. Summarises and clarifies his findings to the patient, describes what next to follow, acknowledges patient and ends encounter politely
18. Presentation of the findings
19. Discussion of the findings and synthesis of findings to make a diagnosis/differential diagnoses
20. Ability to identify normal and abnormal findings, identifies correct findings
21. Ability to identify appropriate investigations in logical sequence
22. Ability to identify appropriate management plan
23. Correct answers to structured questions
24. Global rating: (a) Excellent; (b)Very good or Clear Pass; (c)Bare Pass; (d) Bare Fail; (e) Clear fail; or (f) abysmal
25. Maximum analytical score at this station
26. Candidate's analytical checklist raw score

Appendix 5.2. Performance Descriptors of Physical Examination Skills

In awarding scores for performance at a PE station, the examiners are guided by what are referred to as *performance descriptors*; what qualifies one candidate for a distinction performance and another for a fail. These performance descriptors are shown in Appendix 5.2.

Appendix 5.2. Performance Descriptors (of what you need to do to pass well or fail).

A. EXCELLENT OR OUTSTANDING (SAY MAXIMUM 7 MARKS)
- Faultless physical examination. An exceptional candidate; of a very high standard for their level of studies.
- Demonstrates professional way of eliciting physical signs.
- Identifies physical signs present and does not find clinical signs that are not present.
- Discusses very well, constructs a good differential diagnosis list, and chooses appropriate tests and line of management.

B. Very good or clear pass. Performed at expected level (equivalent to 5 marks)
- Generally admirable performance of PE with only a few minor omissions.
- Presented and discussed well.
- Examiner more than satisfied that candidate deserves a pass at this station.

C. Borderline Pass (equivalent to 4 marks)
- Fairly acceptable performance. A number of faults but none fatal.
- Examiner satisfied that candidate has performed enough to pass.
- Despite some omissions or errors in performance, candidate should be safe to progress.

D. Borderline Fail (equivalent to 3 marks)
- Patchy performance of physical examination. Examiner undecided whether to pass or to fail candidate
- Demonstrated some aspects of the PE; however omissions and inaccuracies equally occurred in performance of the skill.

E. Clear Fail (equivalent to 2 marks)
- Performance of skill did not come up to a passing standard.
- Candidate uses incorrect techniques, omits significant or important tests.
- His general approach is nonprofessional and unsystematic; he is lacking in confidence.
- Missed or misinterpreted signs and/or found signs not present. He is unable to discuss sensibly.
- Not safe to progress.

F. Abysmal fail. (Equivalent to 1 or 0. Could attract negative marks, if allowed)
- Very poor in knowledge and skills.
- Potentially harmful procedures or suggestions.
- Just does not know how to go about the task.
- Performance below expectation even for candidate's juniors.

- Doubtful if candidate attended the course.
- Overall candidate could pose a risk to patient's safety.

Appendix 5.3. Prototype for Starting a Physical Examination Station

An example of starting of candidate-patient encounter at a PES station may run thus:

Candidate to the patient: Good morning Sir, I'm Emeka, a final year medical student in this hospital. I've been asked to examine your chest... Is that okay with you, if I do that?

Patient: No problem

Candidate: Before we continue Sir, may I know your names and age.

Patient: My name is John Jubril, I am forty years old.

Candidate: Thank you Sir. Would you mind taking off your shirt for this examination?

Patient: That's OK. (Removes the shirt, holding it his hands).

Candidate: May I hang the shirt there. And we may use this (drape) to cover you during the examination.

Patient: All right, Doctor

Candidate: I would also like you to be lying with your chest raised like this (adjusts the bed head to cardiac position (30-45°). Are you comfortable?

Patient: It looks OK.

Candidate: Washes their hands. Before we go any further Uncle John, do you have any pain anywhere?

Patient: No.

Candidate to the examiner: Ideally, I would like to expose Mr Jubril's abdomen, chest, and lower limbs, but for the purposes of this examination I will only expose the chest.

On general inspection Mr Jubril looks well, there is no dyspnoea, cyanosis, or any physical discomfort. His hands are warm and well-perfused and there is no clubbing.

On inspection, there is chest asymmetry with a bulge on the left side of the anterior chest.

Et cetera

Appendix 5.4. Potential Favourite Physical Examination Themes

1	Lymphadenopathy	27	Ptosis
2	Male genitalia examination	28	Rectal examination on a plastic model
3	Monocular blindness	29	Renal mass
4	Motor system of the lower limbs	30	Respiratory system examination
5	Motor system of the upper limbs	31	Rheumatoid arthritis
6	Sensory system of the lower limbs	32	Saphena varix
7	Sensory system of the upper limbs	33	Scrubbing up for theatre
8	Multiple sclerosis.	34	Sensorineural hearing loss
9	Muscular back pain	35	Sensory system (upper limbs)
10	Myasthenia gravis	36	Shoulder examination
11	Myopathy	37	Smell and nose examination
12	Nasal polyps	38	Spastic paraparesis
13	Neck examination	39	Speech assessment
14	Neonatal examination	40	Spinal examination
15	Nystagmus	41	Splenomegaly
16	Old tuberculosis	42	Systolic murmur
17	Optic atrophy	43	Thyroglossal cyst
18	Osteoarthritis	44	Simple goitre
19	Papilloedema	45	Thyroid neoplasm
20	Peripheral neuropathy	46	Toxic multiple/diffuse goiter
21	Peripheral vascular disease	47	Toxic/non toxic nodule
22	Pleural effusion	48	Trendelenburg gait
23	Pre-operative assessment	49	Tumours
24	Pseudobulbar palsy	50	Varicose veins
25	Psoriasis	51	Venous insufficiency
26	Psoriatic arthritis	52	Vision and eye examination

EXAMPLES OF CORE ASSESSMENT OBJECTIVES FOR PHYSICAL EXAMINATION STATIONS

Appendix 5 5. Examination of the Cardiovascular Examination I
Candidate Instructions

SCENARIO: Tega Umukoro, m, 40, presents with chest pain worse on walking.

YOUR TASK: Examine the cardiovascular system of Tega Umukoro.

TIME ALLOWED: 5 minutes.

Core Objectives on the Examiner's Rating Scale Would Include that the Candidate:

1. Provides introduction and orientation
2. Establishes rapport with patient
3. Positions and exposes patient appropriately
4. Washes hands
5. Comments on general appearance
6. Inspects praecordium
7. Inspects both hands
8. Determines rate, rhythm, and character of radial pulse
9. *Offers* to record blood pressure
10. Inspects head for signs of anaemia and central cyanosis
11. Assesses jugular venous pressure
12. Assesses character of carotid pulse
13. Determines location and character of apex beat
14. Listens at all four auscultation points
15. Examines the chest
16. Examines and/or offers to examine the abdomen
17. Tests for ankle oedema
18. Palpates peripheral pulses
19. Briefs patient on their findings

EXAMINER: *Please summarise your findings and offer a differential diagnosis.*

20. Accurately summarises key findings
21. Offers appropriate differential diagnosis
22. Candidate's analytical score

23. Global Rating (Fluency of examination and competence in presenting findings, summarizing and forming differential diagnoses)

Appendix 5.6 Examination of the Respiratory System

Candidate Instructions

SCENARIO: This is Mr Everton Wakoma a 52-year-old farmer complaining of shortness of breath and cough.

YOUR TASK: Please examine his respiratory system. Please do a running commentary to the hearing of the examiners.

TIME ALLOWED: 10 minutes.

Core Objectives on the Examiner's Rating Scale Would Include that the Candidate:

1. Introduces self and seeks permission to examine
2. Confirms patient's name and age
3. Asks if patient is currently in any pain
4. Positions patient at 45° and fully exposes chest
5. Washes own hands before examining
6. Counts respiratory rate
7. Inspects hands for clubbing, nicotine staining, and peripheral cyanosis
8. Checks for carbon dioxide retention flap. (Tests for asterixis and beta-agonist tremor)
9. Examines for anaemia and central cyanosis
10. Examines for cervical, supraclavicular, infraclavicular, and axillary lymph nodes
11. Assesses jugular venous pressure
12. Inspects chest for chest movements, scars and deformity (anteriorly and posteriorly)
13. Palpates for tracheal deviation
14. Palpates for character of cardiac apex
15. Palpates for position of cardiac apex
16. Assesses chest expansion
17. Percusses chest
18. Assesses tactile vocal fremitus or vocal resonance

19. Auscultates chest
20. Examines for ankle oedema
21. Offers to measure patient's peak flow
22. Looks into sputum pot
23. Cleans hands by washing or using alcohol gel before and after examination

EXAMINER: *Please summarise your findings and offer a differential diagnosis.*
24. Summarises key findings
25. Offers an appropriate differential diagnosis
26. Candidate's analytical score
27. Global Rating: (Fluency of examination and competence in presenting findings, summarizing and forming differential diagnoses)

Appendix 5.7 Abdominal Examination

Candidate Instructions

SCENARIO
Chief Akpo Kasumi is a 65-year-old gentleman complaining of abdominal swelling.
YOUR TASK: Please examine his gastrointestinal system. Make a running commentary as you proceed.
TIME ALLOWED: 5 minutes

Core Objectives on the Examiner's Rating Scale Would Include that the Candidate:

1. Introduces self and seeks permission to examine
2. Confirms patient's name and age
3. Cleans hands by washing or using alcohol gel
4. Asks if patient is currently in any pain
5. Positions patient supine with one pillow, with abdomen exposed to groin
6. Inspects hands for clubbing, leuconychia, etc
7. Inspects eyes for jaundice and anaemia
8. Palpates for cervical lymphadenopathy (Virchow's node)

9. Inspects trunk (posteriorly and anteriorly) for spider naevi and gynaecomastia
10. Inspects abdomen for scars, distension, masses, dilated abdominal veins and ascites
11. Auscultates for bowel sounds and abdominal aorta bruit
12. Palpates the abdomen, superficial and deep, in all quadrants whilst observing the Face for tenderness
13. Palpates and percusses for hepatomegaly starting in the right iliac fossa
14. Palpates and percusses for splenomegaly starting in the right iliac fossa
15. Ballots both kidneys
16. Palpates and percusses for a distended bladder
17. Palpates the abdominal aorta
18. Inspects and examines the groin for hernias
19. Offers to perform a digital rectal examination and examination of genitalia
20. If appropriate, offers to examine for shifting dullness

EXAMINER: PLEASE SUMMARISE YOUR FINDINGS AND OFFER A DIFFERENTIAL DIAGNOSIS.

21. Summarises key findings
22. Offers an appropriate differential diagnosis
23. Global rating: Fluency of examination and competence in presenting findings, summarizing and forming differential diagnoses
24. Candidate's checklist score

Appendix 5.8 Cardiovascular Disease 2: Acute Chest Pain

Candidate Instructions

SCENARIO: Mr Tames Walker is a 51-year-old bank manager, rushed to the accident and emergency department complaining of acute severe chest pain. He has a long history of hypertension.
YOUR TASK: Examine Mr Walker's cardiovascular system.
TIME ALLOWED: *Five* minutes

PHYSICAL EXAMINATION STATION

Core Objectives on the Examiner's Rating Scale Would Include that the Candidate:

1. Introduces self and seeks permission to examine
2. Confirms patient's name and age
3. Cleans hands by washing or using alcohol gel
4. Asks patient if he is currently in pain and how severe the pain is
5. Positions patient at 45° and drapes with chest exposed
6. Examines hands for clubbing, signs of infective endocarditis, pallor, peripheral cyanosis and capillary refill
7. Assesses radial and carotid pulses (rate, rhythm, character)
8. Offers a blood pressure measurement (you may be told the BP readings)
9. Inspects for anaemia, cyanosis, xanthelasma, and corneal arcus
10. Inspects for a raised JVP
11. Inspects chest for scars and visible apex beat
12. Palpates chest for nature and site of the apex beat, and for any heaves or thrills
13. Auscultates praecordium in all four areas with patient appropriately positioned
14. Auscultates in the left axilla for radiation, and the carotids for radiation/bruits
15. Auscultates the lung bases
16. Palpates the peripheral pulses
17. Feels for sacral and ankle oedema

EXAMINER: PLEASE SUMMARISE YOUR FINDINGS AND OFFER A DIFFERENTIAL DIAGNOSIS.

18. Accurately summarises key findings
19. Offers an appropriate differential diagnosis
20. Global rating: Fluency of examination and competence in presenting findings, summarizing and forming differential diagnoses
21. The station's total analytical score
22. The candidate's total analytical score

Appendix 5.9 Brief Consultation: Thyroid Gland

Candidate Instructions

SCENARIO: At the MOPD a 25-year-old woman presents to you complaining of a neck swelling and weight loss.

YOUR TASK: Please take a short history from her and examine her thyroid gland.

TIME ALLOWED: *Ten* minutes

Core Objectives on the Examiner's Rating Scale Would Include that the Candidate:

1. Introduces self and seeks permission to take a history and examine
2. Ascertains patient's name and age

SHORT HISTORY

3. Establishes how long the swelling has been present and whether it has changed over time
4. Enquires about any local effects of the swelling, in particular pain, difficulty swallowing and difficulty breathing
5. Enquires about systemic effects of thyroid disease – change in weight, preference for hot/cold temperatures, change in bowel habit, lethargy and change in mood
6. Asks if patient is currently in any pain

EXAMINATION

7. Inspects from the end of the bed for signs of thyroid disease
8. Inspects neck from the front and side, commenting on the presence/absence of surgical scars, asymmetry and any obvious swellings
9. Inspects for movement of swelling whilst patient takes a sip of water
10. Palpates swelling
11. Palpates for movement of swelling whilst patient takes a sip of water
12. Palpates for cervical lymphadenopathy
13. Assesses for tracheal deviation
14. Auscultates over swelling for thyroid bruit
15. Measures radial pulse rate

16. Examines hands for sweatiness, palmar erythema, thyroid acropachy and a postural tremor
17. Examines eyes for lid retraction and lag, proptosis and ophthalmoplegia
18. Assesses for proximal myopathy
19. Cleans hands by washing or using alcohol gel

EXAMINER: *PLEASE SUMMARISE YOUR FINDINGS. WHAT IS THE MOST LIKELY DIAGNOSIS?*

20. Accurately summarises key findings
21. Offers an appropriate diagnosis
22. Global rating: Fluency of examination and competence in presenting findings, summarizing and forming differential diagnoses
23. The station's total analytical score
24. The candidate's total analytical score

Appendix 5.10. Examination of the Groin

Candidate Instructions

SCENARIO: Mr Yemi Coker is a 37-year-old bricklayer who complains of a swelling in his groin.

YOUR TASK: To examine his inguinoscrotal region of Mr. Coker.

TIME ALLOWED: *Five* minutes

Core Objectives on the Examiner's Rating Scale Would Include that the Candidate:

1. Introduces self and seeks permission to examine
2. Confirms patient's name and age
3. Cleans hands by washing or using alcohol gel
4. Asks if patient is currently in any pain

PHYSICAL EXAMINATION

5. Stands patient up and exposes groin/scrotum adequately
6. Inspects scrotum
7. Palpates testes, epididymydes and spermatic cords

8. Defines characteristics of scrotal swelling if present (size, shape, fluctuant, transilluminable, cough impulse)
9. Demonstrates inguinal ligament (in relation to pubic tubercle)
10. Examines superficial inguinal rings for a cough impulse
11. Lies patient down
12. If inguinal hernia suspected, assesses whether direct or indirect
13. Palpates femoral arteries, assessing for an aneurysm
14. Examines for inguinal lymphadenopathy
15. Ensures patient is re-clothed. Thanks patient. Explains finding
16. Washes hands again

EXAMINER: *Please summarise your findings. What is the most likely diagnosis?*

17. Accurately summarises key findings
18. Offers an appropriate diagnosis
19. Global rating: Fluency of examination and competence in presenting findings, summarizing and forming differential diagnoses
20. Station's total analytical score
21. The candidate's total analytical score

Appendix 5.11. Examination of the Venous System of the Lower Limbs

Candidate Instructions

SCENARIO: Mrs Alice Romberg is a 38- year-old teacher who complains of painful "veins or nerves"

YOUR TASK: To examine her legs with respect to the venous system.

TIME ALLOWED: 5 minutes.

Core Objectives on the Examiner's Rating Scale Would Include that the Candidate:

1. Introduces self and seeks permission to examine
2. Confirms patient's name and age
3. Cleans hands by washing or using alcohol gel
4. Asks patient about site and degree of pain
5. Asks if patient is currently in any pain

6. Adequately exposes both legs with the patient standing up
7. Inspects both legs (compares for shape; and comments on the presence/absence of previous surgery, skin changes above the medial malleolus and distribution of varicosities, including a saphena varix in the groin)
8. Assesses the temperature of both lower limbs
9. Assesses for tenderness and palpates along the medial side of the lower leg
10. Palpates the sapheno-femoral junction for a cough impulse (suggestive of sapheno-femoral incompetence)
11. If a saphena varix is present, palpates it for a cough impulse
12. Performs the tap test (a percussion impulse is suggestive of incompetence in the superficial veins)
13. Performs the Trendelenburg test (if the veins are controlled by a tourniquet or fingers at the sapheno-femoral junction, this is suggestive of sapheno-femoral incompetence)
14. If the Trendelenburg test is negative, performs the tourniquet test to find the level at which venous incompetence lies
15. Auscultates for a bruit over marked venous clusters
16. Examines the peripheral pulses (femoral, popliteal, dorsalis pedis and posterior tibial)
17. Cleans hands again by washing or using alcohol gel
18. Properly brings the patient encounter to a close

EXAMINER: *Please summarise your findings. What is the most likely diagnosis?*

19. Accurately summarises key findings
20. Offers the correct most likely diagnosis.
21. Examiner's global rating (Global Rating: Fluency of examination Competence in presenting findings, summarizing and forming differential diagnoses)
22. Station's total analytical score
23. The candidate's total analytical score

OSCE Skills for Trainees in Medicine

Appendix 5.12 Brief Consultation: Bedside Diagnosis of Peripheral Arterial Disease

Candidate Instructions

SCENARIO: Mr Tom Tanga is a 68-year-old man with diabetes mellitus of 10 years. He is complaining of pain on walking.

YOUR TASK: Please take a brief history and examine his peripheral vascular system, concentrating on his lower limbs.

TIME ALLOWED: Ten minutes

Core Objectives on the Examiner's Rating Scale Would Include that the Candidate:

BRIEF HISTORY
1. Introduces self and seeks permission to examine
2. Confirms patient's name and age
3. Asks about duration of pain
4. Asks about onset and severity of pain
5. Asks about relieving and aggravating factors
6. Asks about associated features such as chest pain, hypertension

PHYSICAL EXAMINATION
7. Transits smoothly
8. Cleans hands by washing or using alcohol gel
9. Exposes lower limbs adequately
10. Asks whether patient is in pain
11. Inspects for ischaemic skin changes, ulcers and surgical scars (looks especially for ulcers on the tips of the toes and around the heels)
12. Assesses the temperature of both legs
13. Checks for capillary refilling time
14. Feels for pulses: femoral, popliteal, posterior tibial and dorsalis pedis
15. Auscultates for bruits (femoral and popliteal)
16. Assesses for venous guttering (elevates the leg to approximately 15°)
17. Checks for Buerger's angle (the angle at which the leg becomes pale)

18. Performs Buerger's test (after checking Buerger's angle, asks the patient to hang his legs over the side of the bed – looks for reactive hyperaemia)
19. States intention to examine the rest of the peripheral vascular system
20. States intention to examine the heart
21. States intention to perform an ankle–brachial pressure index (ABPI) reading using Hand-held Doppler
22. Cleans hands again by washing or using alcohol gel
23. Closes the encounter appropriately

EXAMINER: *Please summarise your findings. What is the most likely diagnosis and how will you confirm it?*

24. Accurately summarises key findings
25. Offers the correct most likely diagnosis and a confirmatory test.
26. Examiner's global rating (Global Rating: Fluency of examination, competence in presenting findings, summarizing and forming differential diagnoses)
27. Station's total analytical score
28. The candidate's total analytical score

Appendix 5.13 Neurological Examination of the Lower Limbs

Candidate Instructions

SCENARIO: Mr Tahu Tetoro is a 50-year-old man who had a stroke about a year ago. He complains of weakness in his right leg.
YOUR TASK: To examine Tahu's lower limbs neurologically; (limit your examination to the motor system).
TIME ALLOWED: Five minutes

Core Objectives on the Examiner's Rating Scale Would Include that the Candidate:

1. Introduces self and seeks permission to examine
2. Confirms patient's name and age
3. Cleans hands by washing or using alcohol gel
4. Asks if patient is currently in any pain
5. Positions patient appropriately, exposing both lower limbs

6. Inspects lower limbs – looking for wasting and fasciculation
7. Assesses the lower limbs for tone, including testing for ankle clonus if tone is increased
8. Tests power of hip flexion
9. Tests power of hip extension
10. Tests power of knee flexion
11. Tests power of knee extension
12. Tests power of ankle dorsiflexion
13. Tests power of plantar flexion
14. Tests power of eversion of forefoot
15. Tests power of inversion of forefoot
16. Assesses reflexes (knee, ankle and plantar) with reinforcement if necessary
17. Tests heel–shin coordination
18. Observes gait– comments on posture, arm swing, step size and equality, ataxia and circumduction
19. Performs Romberg's test
20. Cleans hands by washing or using alcohol gel
21. Closes the encounter appropriately

EXAMINER: *Please summarise your findings. What is the most likely diagnosis and how will you confirm it?*

22. Accurately summarises key findings
23. Offers the most likely diagnosis and its confirmation.
24. Station's total analytical score
25. Candidate's analytical score
26. Global Rating: (Fluency of examination and competence in presenting findings, summarizing and forming differential diagnoses)

Appendix 5.14. Short Consultation: Evaluation of Unsteady Walking

Candidate Instructions

SCENARIO: Mrs Babara Tatata, a 70-year-old retired magistrate is complaining of being unsteady whilst walking.

YOUR TASK: Please carry out a neurological examination to assess her balance and cerebellar function.

TIME ALLOWED: **Ten** minutes.

PHYSICAL EXAMINATION STATION

Core Objectives on the Examiner's Rating Scale Would Include that the Candidate:
1. Introduces self and seeks permission to examine
2. Confirms patient's name and age
3. Enquires about relevant symptoms
4. Cleans hands by washing or using alcohol gel
5. Asks if patient is currently in any pain
6. Stands at the end of the bed and observes for presence of wheelchair, urinary catheter, titibulation
7. Examines for nystagmus
8. Assesses for dysarthric speech (asks patient to say 'British constitution' or 'baby hippopotamus')
9. Assesses tone in upper limbs
10. Asks patient to perform finger–nose test, looking for upper limb ataxia
11. Assesses for dysdiadochokinesis (by observing rapid alternating hand movements)
12. Examines fine finger movements (asks patient to oppose each finger in turn against her thumb)
13. Assesses for cerebellar drift
14. Asks patient to perform heel–shin test, looking for lower limb ataxia
15. Assesses gait
16. Assesses tandem gait (asks patient to walk heel to toe)
17. Performs Romberg's test
18. Cleans hands again by washing or using alcohol gel
19. Closes the encounter appropriately

EXAMINER: *Please summarise your findings. Tell us the most likely differential diagnosis and one confirmatory test for it.*
20. Accurately summarises key findings
21. Offers the correct most likely differential diagnosis and a confirmatory test.
22. Station's total checklist score
23. Candidate's checklist score
24. Global Rating: (Fluency of examination and competence in presenting findings, summarizing and forming differential diagnoses)

Appendix 5.15. Eye Examination

Candidate Instructions

SCENARIO: Mr Deedo Gooseman is a 22-year-old student who complains of double vision.
YOUR TASK: To examine Mr. Gooseman's eyes
TIME ALLOWED 10 minutes

Core Objectives on the Examiner's Rating Scale Would Include that the Candidate:

1. Introduces self and seeks permission to examine
2. Confirms patient's name and age
3. Enquires about relevant symptoms – diplopia, visual field loss
4. Cleans hands by washing or using alcohol gel
5. Asks if patient is currently in any pain
6. Positions patient appropriately
7. Inspects for ptosis, squint, exophthalmos and pupil size and irregularity
8. Enquires about and tests for visual acuity (uses Snellen chart if one is available); otherwise asks patient to read ordinary type face/count fingers.(visual acuity should be tested with spectacles or contact lenses if usually worn by the patient)
9. States intention to test colour vision using Ishihara colour plates
10. Assesses visual neglect (crude test for visual field loss)
11. Examines visual fields carefully (tests for a peripheral defect and uses red hat pin to delineate the patient's blind spot and any scotomas, and to test for macular sparing)
12. Examines eye movements vertically and horizontally (enquires about diplopia and observes for nystagmus)
13. Examines for pupillary light and accommodation reflexes
14. Sets and handles ophthalmoscope correctly
15. Assesses for a red reflex with the ophthalmoscope
16. Shows correct technique for viewing fundi
17. Shows correct technique for viewing discs
18. Cleans hands again by washing or using alcohol gel
19. Closes the encounter appropriately

EXAMINER: *Please summarise your findings. What is the most likely diagnosis and how will you confirm it?*
20. Summarises the key findings
21. Offers an appropriate list of differential diagnosis and a confirmatory test.
22. Station's total analytical score
23. Candidate's analytical score
24. Global Rating: (Fluency of examination and competence in presenting findings, summarizing and forming differential diagnoses)

Appendix 5.16. Assessment of Difficulty in Hearing

Candidate Instructions

SCENARIO: Mr Duro Swe is a 62-year-old man who presents with difficulty in hearing
YOUR TASK: Please assess Mr Swe's hearing.
TIME ALLOWED: Five minutes.

Core Objectives on the Examiner's Rating Scale Would Include that the Candidate:

1. Introduces self and seeks permission to take a history and examine
2. Confirms patient's name and age

HISTORY
3. Establishes onset and duration of hearing loss
4. Establishes whether patient has had previous ENT surgery
5. Establishes whether one or both ears are affected
6. Establishes whether hearing loss is to high-pitched or low-pitched sounds
7. Establishes severity of hearing loss and impact on patient's life
8. Enquires about associated symptoms – vertigo and tinnitus, discharge, loss of balance, pain
9. Enquires about possible causal factors – noise exposure, treatment with ototoxic drugs, family history

EXAMINATION
10. Cleans hands by washing or using alcohol gel
11. Asks if patient is currently in any pain
12. Tests hearing in each ear using speech
13. Performs the Rinne test using a 512 Hz tuning fork
14. Performs the Weber test using a 512 Hz tuning fork
15. Inspects outer ears and behind the ears for any abnormalities and surgical scars
16. Holds otoscope and patient's ear correctly
17. Inspects ear canals (otitis externa, wax)
18. Inspects tympanic membranes and identifies normal or abnormal anatomy
19. Cleans hands again by washing or using alcohol gel
20. Closes the encounter appropriately

EXAMINER: *Please summarise your findings and offer a differential diagnosis and further tests.*
21. Summarises key findings
22. Offers an appropriate list of differential diagnosis and further relevant tests.
23. Station's total analytical score
24. Candidate's analytical score
25. Global Rating: (Fluency of examination and competence in presenting findings, summarizing and forming differential diagnoses)

Appendix 5.17. Brief Consultation: Skin History and Examination

Candidate Instructions

SCENARIO: You are the JR in the GOPD when Miss Louisa Brown, a 38-year-old secretary, presents complaining of a rash she has had for about two months now.

YOUR TASK: To take a short history from her and examine her skin.

TIME ALLOWED: **Five** minutes

PHYSICAL EXAMINATION STATION

Core Objectives on the Examiner's Rating Scale Would Include that the Candidate:

1. Introduces self and seeks permission to take a history and examine
2. Confirms patient's name and age

HISTORY

3. Enquires about onset and duration of rash, establishing whether it has changed over time
4. Establishes site of rash
5. Establishes associated symptoms – itchiness, discharge and pain/tenderness
6. Enquires about precipitating/relieving factors including previous treatment
7. Establishes impact of rash on patient and lifestyle
8. Enquires about allergies
9. Enquires about any problems with joints
10. Establishes patient's past medical and drug history
11. Asks if patient is currently in any pain

EXAMINATION

12. Cleans hands by washing or using alcohol gel
13. Inspects skin, nails, and joints appropriately
14. Describes any nail/joint pathology
15. Palpates rash
16. Describes distribution and morphology of rash
17. Cleans hands again by washing or using alcohol gel
18. Closes the encounter appropriately

EXAMINER: PLEASE SUMMARISE YOUR FINDINGS OF THE CASE AND OFFER A DIFFERENTIAL DIAGNOSIS.

19. Summarises key findings
20. Offers an appropriate list of differential diagnosis
21. Station's total analytical score
22. Candidate's analytical score
23. Global Rating: (Fluency of examination and competence in presenting findings, summarizing and forming differential diagnoses)

Appendix 5.18. Examination of a Mass

Candidate Instructions

SCENARIO: Mrs Titi Koruma is 34 years old. She has come to the SOP complaining of a swelling on her right thigh.

YOUR TASK: To examine the lump on Mrs Koruma's thigh.

TIME ALLOWED: Five minutes

Core Objectives on the Examiner's Rating Scale Would Include that the Candidate:

1. Establishes rapport: Greets patient. Introduces self. Explains purpose of encounter and seeks consent
2. Confirms patient's name, demographics, and occupation
3. Ensures patient's comfort and modesty; asks about pain
4. Cleans hands by washing or using alcohol gel
5. Inspects lump and overlying skin
6. **Palpates lump and assesses**:
   a. temperature
   b. size
   c. shape
   d. surface
   e. consistency
   f. mobility
   g. Transilluminates lump

7. Assesses whether lump is pulsatile
8. Examines or indicates need to examine inguinal lymph nodes
9. Cleans hands again by washing or using alcohol gel
10. Closes the encounter appropriately

EXAMINER: PLEASE SUMMARISE YOUR FINDINGS AND OFFER A DIFFERENTIAL DIAGNOSIS.

11. Summarises key findings
12. Offers an appropriate differential diagnosis
13. Station's total analytical score
14. Candidate's analytical score
15. Global Rating: (Fluency of examination and competence in presenting findings, summarizing and forming differential diagnoses)

6

Practical Procedure Skills Station

6.1. Practical Procedures in Clinical Medicine

6.2. Categories of Practical Procedure Stations

6.3. Elements at a Practical Procedure Station

6.4. Advice on Practical Procedure Skills Station

6.5. Examples of Practical Procedure Stations

6.6. Chapter Six Summary.

6.7. Chapter Six Recap Exercises

6.8. Bibliography and Resources

6.9. Appendices

OSCE Skills for Trainees in Medicine

6.1. PRACTICAL PROCEDURES IN CLINICAL MEDICINE

Technical skills are frequently required of doctors and other healthcare workers to execute practical diagnostic and therapeutic procedures. Such procedures are not usually directly assessed in traditional clinical examinations. The practical procedure skills (PPS) station in an OSCE provides an opportunity to assess such skills. At a PPS station a student is given a technical task relevant to clinical practice to perform while the examiner observes and rates their performance.

6.2 CATEGORIES OF PRACTICAL PROCEDURE STATIONS

The principal use of a practical procedure skills station in OSCE is the testing of the candidate's psychomotor skills and to some extent their knowledge of the procedure and how they communicate with the patient as they perform the procedure. You may also be asked to demonstrate the use of an instrument or equipment at a practical procedure station.

The practical procedures expected to be performed by students during their undergraduate and/or postgraduate training include but not limited to the following:

- Abdominal paracentesis
- Administering i.v. drugs
- Administration of oxygen therapy
- Arterial line placement
- Arterial puncture
- Arterial puncture for ABG
- Arthrocentesis
- Cardiopulmonary resuscitation
- Central line placement
- Collection of midstream urine
- CVP measurement
- Direct cardioversion
- Establishment of i.v access using a giving set
- Faecal occult blood testing
- Flexible sigmoidoscopy
- Interpretation of charts
- Male and female urinary catheterisation
- Measurement of anthropometry
- Measurement of blood glucose, POC
- Measurement of blood pressure
- Measurement of body temperature
- Measurement of peak expiratory flow rate
- Measurement of transcutaneous O2 saturation
- Nasogastric tube placement
- Performance and/or interpretation of a 12 lead ECG
- Performing a blood culture
- Pregnancy testing

Scrubbing up and gowning for surgical/ and sterile procedures
Skin biopsies and shavings
Skin suturing
Thoracentesis
Urinalysis using Multistix
Venepuncture

The above are the types of tasks that may feature in an OSCE Practical Procedure Station.

6.3. ELEMENTS AT A PRACTICAL PROCEDURE STATION

There are two main elements you are likely to meet at a PPS station: a group of examination staff with their assistants and a set of materials/equipment and information items.

Staff at a Practical Procedure Station

An examiner or rater will be present at a PPS station but only some stations need the presence of an assistant, a technician, an SP, and/or a station time keeper. The examiner/rater may be a teacher in the specialty, some other health professional, or a technical person such as a technologist. Whoever the rater is, give them due recognition and respect as you would to your own teachers.

Information Elements at a Practical Procedure Station

At the practical procedure skills (PPS) station you will be presented with a set of documents and instructions describing what is to be done and how it should be done. Most PPS stations will provide the following information items for your attention: *Station Number, Station Title, Station Construct or Purpose, Time Allowed, Scenario or Stem to the Question. and Instructions for the Candidate*. Depending on the task, other information may include technician and patient instructions. Of all these, what concerns you the candidate most will be the *Candidate Instructions*.

The *Candidate Instruction* would include the *Time Allowed* to perform the task; which is clearly stated, usually about 3-5 minutes for undergraduate examinations and much longer for postgraduate examinations. A description of the case scenario or stem to the question will usually precede what task has been cut out for you.

Information and Instructions for the Candidate

The instructions to the candidates usually give:

SCENARIO: States who you (the candidate) are and the setting of the problem. e.g. You are the pathology registrar to whom a CSF sample from a child with acute fever has been sent.

YOUR TASK: The task to be undertaken by you, e.g. Please examine and report on the CSF slide from a patient with fever.

TIME ALLOWED: You have 3 or 5 minutes for this task.

FURTHER INSTRUCTIONS: Further instruction or information may be given to you (such as… examiners will ask you some questions; to take notes; and whether information will be used at the next station).

Information for the Patient at a Practical Procedure Station

A patient at a PPS station may be real but usually simulators are used. Real patient involvement is more limited at a PPS station than at a clinical OSCE station. Such simulated patients would mostly be used to obtain measurements such as lung function test, BP, and ECG tracing. Relate to the simulated patient or actor as you would to a real patient. If using mannequins or anatomical models, tell the examiners how you would have treated a patient in similar circumstances.

Materials at a Practical Procedure Station

The materials at a practical procedure station will depend on the station purpose and task. You may find a trolley or tray with the usual ward or clinic equipment all available. What to use or ask for may be left to you. You must become familiar with such equipment and know their indications and how to use them during your training. Be familiar with the common potential procedures and determine what type of information and equipment (Figure 6.1) you would need to perform each task.

PRACTICAL PROCEDURE STATION

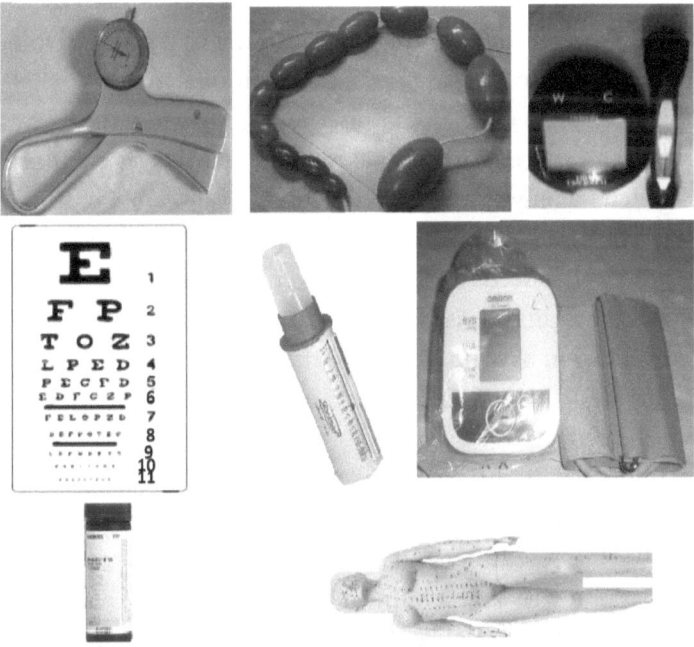

Figure 6.1. A Variety of Instruments and Devices May Be Placed at a Practical Procedure Station. *Such devices tend to be portable and the ones you must have been using in your training.*

Similar to the OSCE physical examination station, most of what you need at the PPS station should be provided but you can bring along your own stethoscope, flash light, and ophthalmoscope. You may be more at home using your usual equipment.

6.4. ADVICE ON PRACTICAL PROCEDURE SKILLS STATION

1. Expectations of the examiners about your performance at a practical procedure skills station are similar to those at a manned clinical station especially when a patient is present. However, unlike clinical manned stations, you need not struggle with eliciting and interpreting symptoms and signs or making a diagnosis at a PP station. What is required of you is a demonstration of what you have (supposedly) been doing all along during your training.

2. To do well at a PPS station, you would have practised the common tasks several times during your training or postings. Doing it the first time under examination conditions could be challenging and agonising. To maximise your returns at the PPS station, the procedure must be fluently and confidently performed; this generally only comes from practice.
3. If you have a skills' centre this is where you can perfect your practical procedure skills using manikins and models. Practise as a group and reverse roles as candidates and examiners or SPs.
4. Even if you have no access to a skills centre, start from somewhere (besides patients) and then transfer the skills to the clinic or the ward setting.
5. Some of the practical skills stations are difficult to complete in the short time given in an OSCE setting. You need to have mastered the skill to be able to carry it out fluently and satisfactorily in the time allocated in OSCE/OSPE setting. Therefore, internalise the lists of equipment and the steps for each of the common practical skills for your level, they will then become second nature to you.
6. Remember to always confirm the "patient's" identity, even if a role player or a manikin is being used. Ensure that you establish rapport with your "patient", explain the indication and procedure, and seek their permission, giving them an opportunity to express any concerns. If using a manikin or a model, tell the examiner how would go about it, were it a real patient.
7. The examiner may ask you some questions at the end of the procedure or why you would want to do certain things; be prepared to answer confidently. If you are unable to answer the question, do not be downcast as there are other aspects you could have done well.
8. Make serious efforts to be proficient at the frequently featured tasks at a PPS station such as the following:

Abdominal paracentesis
Administering i.v. drugs
Administration of oxygen therapy
Basic life support
Cardiopulmonary resuscitation
Collection of midstream urine
Demonstration of skills using simulators and models
Establishment of i.v access using a giving set
Examining slides using a microscope
Faecal occult blood testing
Interpretation of charts
Interpreting images such as X-rays, CT scans, USS
Interpreting lab data results
Lumbar puncture
Measurement of blood pressure
Measurement of body temperature
Measurement of capillary blood glucose
Measurement of height and weight
Measurement of peak expiratory flow rate
Measurement of transcutaneous O_2 saturation
Measuring and recording peripheral pulses
Nasogastric tube placement
Performance/or interpretation of a 12-lead ECG
Performing a blood culture
Pregnancy testing
Scrubbing up and gowning for surgical and sterile procedures
Skin biopsies and shavings
Skin suturing
Urinalysis using test strips
Urinary catheterisation
Venepuncture

6.5. EXAMPLES OF PRACTICAL PROCEDURE SKILLS STATIONS

We shall use two common procedures, measuring a blood pressure and providing basic life support, to illustrate how a PPS station is run.

6.5.1. Measuring Blood Pressure

General Information about the Station

All those involved about this station should note the following body of information:

STATION NUMBER: 10

Table 6.1. Rating Scale Assessment for Blood Pressure Measurement

Scoring: Very good, 5; Good, 4; Average, 3; Poor, 2; Very poor, 1; Not done 0. Please circle your awarded scores

	Task component/ item	Score
1	Greets patient. Introduces self. Obtains patient's demographics. Uses patient's surname. Explains purpose. Seeks consent. (0-1-2-3-4-5)	
2	Establishes rapport (at start and throughout the process) and makes the patient at ease (0-1-2-3-4-5)	
3	Selects/comments on appropriate cuff size bladder (i.e. width >40% and length > 80% of arm circumference) (0-1-2-3-4-5)	
4	Checks functionality of equipment. (0-1-2-3-4-5)	
5	Elicits how long patient has rested and about eating, drinking caffeine, smoking or exercising 30 min before (0-1-2-3-4-5)	
6	Positions patient and equipment appropriately. (0-1-2-3-4-5)	
7	Gets patient comfortably seated, legs uncrossed, with feet flat on floor, back supported for a period of rest. (0-1-2-3-4-5)	
8	Exposes the arms and removes any restrictions Supports arm at the level of patient's heart. (0-1-2-3-4-5)	
9	Ensures that manometer is upright and at eye level. (0-1-2-3-4-5)	
10	Palpates both radial pulses (0-1-2-3-4-5)	
11	Palpates a brachial artery and wraps cuff smoothly and snugly around patient's arm, with the lower edge about 3 cm above elbow crease (0-1-2-3-4-5)	
12	Ensures that the sphyg is at heart level. Inflates the cuff, determines rough SBP by palpating the radial or brachial artery having forewarned patient of slight discomfort. (0-1-2-3-4-5)	
13	Deflates cuff, applies diaphragm of stethoscope, and re-inflates the cuff to 20 - 30 mmHg above palpated SBP. (0-1-2-3-4-5)	
14	Deflates cuff slowly (2 -3 mm per second) until SBP and DBP recorded while listening (0-1-2-3-4-5)	
15	Deflates cuff fully after each reading (0-1-2-3-4-5)	
16	Repeats (or requests to repeat) measurement in same position after at least two minutes. (0-1-2-3-4-5)	
17	Repeats (or requests to repeat the measurement on the opposite arm). Decides on which arm to use. (0-1-2-3-4-5)	

Table 6.1. Rating Scale Assessment for Blood Pressure Measurement

Scoring: Very good, 5; Good, 4; Average, 3; Poor, 2; Very poor, 1; Not done 0. Please circle your awarded scores

Task component/ item	Score
18 Repeats (or requests to repeat after 2 minutes of standing) the BP measurement. Ensures that manometer remains at heart level, with the help of a station assistant. (0-1-2-3-4-5)	
19 Removes sphygmomanometer, folds, and replaces in container. (0-1-2-3-4-5)	
20 Tells, or hands over to the patient the written BP readings (0-1-2-3-4-5)	
21 Thanks the patient and addresses any of the patient's concerns or questions regarding the BP measurement. (0-1-2-3-4-5)	
22 Explains manoeuvres clearly, transitions smoothly; allows patient to accommodate. (0-1-2-3-4-5)	
Examiner: Comment on the BP	
23 Answers to Questions (0-1-2-3-4-5)	
24 Global rating: (A) Excellent; (B) Very good; (C) Good; (D) Borderline pass; (E) borderline fail; (F) Abysmal fail	
25 General Comments on candidate or station	
Name Signature Date	

STATION TITLE: Practical Procedure Station

STATION CONSTRUCT: The purpose of this station is to test the candidate's ability to accurately measure a blood pressure in an adult.

SCENARIO: Mr. Luka Kpado has been receiving treatment for essential hypertension for the last five years. He was last seen at the clinic over a year ago. He maintains that he has been faithfully taking his medications.

TIME ALLOWED: Five minutes

Information and Instructions for Candidate

CLINICAL SCENARIO: You are a house officer working with a medical consultant. The patient described above is at the MOP for a follow-up visit after a long absence.

YOUR TASK: To accurately measure his blood pressure using the materials and equipment provided. You should do a running commentary to the hearing of the examiners who will also ask you a few questions.
TIME ALLOWED: 5 minutes

Information and Instructions for the Station Examiner
- Please read the general information about this station. The candidate is a final year medical student. Please award marks for each component of the procedure as in Table 6.1. In addition to rating performance on individual task components, you are to grade the overall performance of the candidate. This global rating should be *independent of your analytical scores* of the candidate at this station.

6.5.2. Practical Procedure Station: Basic Life Support

General Information about the Station
All those concerned with this station should note the following body of information and instructions:

STATION NUMBER: 14
STATION TITLE: Practical Procedure Station
STATION CONSTRUCT: The purpose of this station is to test the candidate's ability to perform basic life support outside the hospital environment.
TIME ALLOWED: Five minutes
SCENARIO: Mr Daniel Davies, a 45-year-old attorney is found collapsed near the toilet in the court premises.

Information and Instructions for the Candidate
SCENARIO: You are a medical practitioner who is visiting the High Court. You find a man Mr Daniel Davies, a 45-year-old attorney, collapsed near the toilet in the court premises.
YOUR TASK: Using the materials (including a manikin [to represent Mr Davies]) provided, assess Mr Davies and react as appropriate. You are to provide a running commentary as you proceed.

PRACTICAL PROCEDURE STATION

TIME ALLOWED: You have 5 minutes to complete the procedure.

Information and Instructions for the Station Examiner

Please read the general information and instructions to the candidate at this station. The candidate is a junior resident. Please award marks for each component of the procedure as indicated below for performance on *Adult BLS Skills: One-Man Rescuer, Outside Hospital.*

In addition to rating the performance on individual task components, you are to grade the overall performance of the candidate. This global rating should be *independent* of your checklist scores for the candidate at this station. Please do not discuss your scores with your co-examiner.

The candidate:

(Item scoring descriptors: Excellent, 4; Good, 3; Average, 2; Poor, 1; Very poor or not done, 0.)

I. Assesses for any danger in the situation either for himself or the patient. (0-1-2-3-4)

II. Checks if there is any response from the patient (gently shakes the patient's shoulders and loudly shouts into both ears asking them their name and 'Can you hear me?' (0-1-2-3-4)

III. If there is no response, shouts for help or calls the ambulance service. (0-1-2-3)

IV. Opens patient's airway using the head tilt, chin lift technique. (0-1-2-3-4)

V. Ensures that there is no physical blockage by the tongue, vomit or anything else. (0-1-2-3-4)

VI. Checks the patient's breathing and circulation simultaneously. (0-1-2-3)

VII. Kneels by the side of the victim

VIII. Checks the patient's breathing (5-10 seconds); maintains the head tilt and jaw thrust, places his face and ear over the mouth to feel for any respiratory effort whilst observing the chest for any movement. (0-1-2-3-4)

IX. Simultaneous to Step VIII, places his two fingers over the carotid pulse to assess circulation. (0-1-2-3)

OSCE Skills for Trainees in Medicine

X. Breathing and/or circulation absent, calls for help appropriately. (0-1-2-3)

XI. Starts chest compressions. Places one hand over the sternum roughly in the middle, interlocks his fingers and positions himself vertically above his hands. (0-1-2-3-4)

XII. Places the index finger of one hand next to the sternal notch. Places the heel of the palm of the other hand on the lower half of the sternum next to the index finger. Places the heel of the first hand on top of the second. Interlocks the fingers of both hands and lifts the fingers off the chest wall. Straightens both elbows and locks them into position. Positions his shoulders directly over the victim's chest, using his body weight to compress the victim's sternum. (0-1-2-3-4-5)

XIII. Depresses the sternum 4-5 cm and releases the pressure. Repeats this 30 times at a rate of 80-100 per minute. (0-1-2-3-4)

XIV. Then starts a combination of 2 rescue breaths and 30 chest compressions. (0-1-2-3-4)

XV. With the head tilt and jaw thrust in place, pinches the soft part of the nose so that it is closed, opens his mouth, seal his lips around theirs and blows steadily for 2 seconds. (0-1-2-3-4)

XVI. Watches the chest to check that it rises and falls with the breath. (0-1-2-3)

XVII. Returns from giving the breaths to give 30 chest compressions. (0-1-2-3-4)

XVIII. Tells examiners when to stop (continue until either further help arrives, the patient regains consciousness or he can no longer physically continue). (0-1-2-3-4)

XIX *Global rating:* **Clear pass, 4; Borderline pass, 3; Borderline fail, 2; Clear fail, 1**.

XX *Maximum total analytical score*

XXI *Candidate's total analytical Score*

(Item scoring descriptors: Excellent, 4; Good, 3; Average, 2; Poor, 1; Very poor or not done, 0.)

I. Assesses for any danger in the situation either for himself or the patient. (0-1-2-3-4)

II. Checks if there is any response from the patient (gently shakes the patient's shoulders and loudly shouts into both ears asking them their name and 'Can you hear me?' (0-1-2-3-4)

III.	If there is no response, shouts for help or calls the ambulance service. (0-1-2-3)
IV.	Opens patient's airway using the head tilt, chin lift technique. (0-1-2-3-4)
V.	Ensures that there is no physical blockage by the tongue, vomit or anything else. (0-1-2-3-4)
VI.	Checks the patient's breathing and circulation simultaneously. (0-1-2-3)
VII.	Kneels by the side of the victim
VIII.	Checks the patient's breathing (5-10 seconds); maintains the head tilt and jaw thrust, places his face and ear over the mouth to feel for any respiratory effort whilst observing the chest for any movement. (0-1-2-3-4)
IX.	Simultaneous to Step VIII, places his two fingers over the carotid pulse to assess circulation. (0-1-2-3)
X.	Breathing and/or circulation absent, calls for help appropriately. (0-1-2-3)
XI.	Starts chest compressions. Places one hand over the sternum roughly in the middle, interlocks his fingers and positions himself vertically above his hands. (0-1-2-3-4)
XII.	Places the index finger of one hand next to the sternal notch. Places the heel of the palm of the other hand on the lower half of the sternum next to the index finger. Places the heel of the first hand on top of the second. Interlocks the fingers of both hands and lifts the fingers off the chest wall. Straightens both elbows and locks them into position. Positions his shoulders directly over the victim's chest, using his body weight to compress the victim's sternum. (0-1-2-3-4-5)
XIII.	Depresses the sternum 4-5 cm and releases the pressure. Repeats this 30 times at a rate of 80-100 per minute. (0-1-2-3-4)
XIV.	Then starts a combination of 2 rescue breaths and 30 chest compressions. (0-1-2-3-4)
XV.	With the head tilt and jaw thrust in place, pinches the soft part of the nose so that it is closed, opens his mouth, seal his lips around theirs and blows steadily for 2 seconds. (0-1-2-3-4)
XVI.	Watches the chest to check that it rises and falls with the breath. (0-1-2-3)
XVII.	Returns from giving the breaths to give 30 chest compressions. (0-1-2-3-4)

XVIII.	Tells examiners when to stop (continue until either further help arrives, the patient regains consciousness or he can no longer physically continue). (0-1-2-3-4)	
XIX	Global rating: Clear pass, 4; Borderline pass, 3; Borderline fail, 2; Clear fail, 1.	
XX	Maximum total analytical score	
XXI	Candidate's total analytical Score	

Note that basic life support is one of the most important skills you must acquire at the medical school and as such you are likely to be examined on this station regularly. So make sure you master it thoroughly! You may download videos to aid your practice. See also the appendices for another example.

6.6. CHAPTER SIX SUMMARY
- Practical procedure skills (PPS) stations enable examiners to assess technical skills required of doctors and other healthcare workers to execute diagnostic and therapeutic procedures.
- Practical Procedure Skills stations are manned and scored using a checklist or a rating scale.
- Simulated patients, instruments, models, and manikins may be made use of to carry out the tasks at PPS stations.
- If you aspire to do well at a PPS station, you should practise the common diagnostic and therapeutic procedures several times and be familiar with the common equipment and instruments needed to execute the tasks.

6.7. CHAPTER SIX RECAP EXERCISES
Let us recap what we have discussed in this chapter by answering the following quizzes:
1. List three materials that you may find at a Practical Procedure Skills Station.
2. List five procedures that you are very familiar with and which are potential tasks for a practical procedure station.
3. List the major steps in performing a basic life support in a hospital setting.
4. List five common mistakes that you think (from your practice sessions) that candidates often make at PPS stations.

PRACTICAL PROCEDURE STATION

5. List the equipment and materials you would need to perform the following procedures:
   a. Delivery of oxygen
   b. Giving blood transfusion
   c. Setting up a CVP measurement
   d. Running an ECG tracing
   e. Female bladder catheterisation

6. Which three procedures do you think each of the following groups of doctors must know well and deserve to be in an OSCE exercise?
   a. A preregistration house officer
   b. A Registrar in Obstetrics & Gynaecology
   c. A Senior Registrar in Cardiology

6.8. BIBLIOGRAPHY AND RESOURCES. See page 249

6.9. APPENDICES

Appendix 6.1. Basic Life Support Station: In-Hospital Scenario

Candidate Instructions

SCENARIO: The ward sister phones you, the medical registrar on call that Mr James Gadomu Hussein, a man recovering from acute myocardial infarction on ward E5 has collapsed.

YOUR TASK: Given the clinical scenario, take appropriate action. Make a running commentary to the hearing of the examiners. A manikin and other resuscitation materials are provided.

TIME ALLOWED: Five minutes.

(Scoring: Not done/ poorly done, 0; adequately done 1).

Core Items on the Examiner's Rating Scale Would Include that the Candidate:

1.	Demonstrates a safe approach (for self or 'patient')	0 – 1
2.	Shouts for help	0 – 1
3.	Checks patient for a response	0 – 1
4.	Turns patient onto back	0 – 1

5.	Opens airway using head-tilt, chin-lift technique	0 – 1
6.	Looks into the mouth	0 – 1
7.	Listens, feels, and looks for breathing	0 – 1
8.	Assesses carotid pulse	0 – 1
9.	Ensures that resuscitation team is called	0 – 1
10.	Delivers 30 chest compressions	0 – 1
11.	Aims for a rate of 100 compressions per minute	0 – 1
12.	Aims to depress sternum by 4–5 cm	0 – 1
14.	Secures airway	0 – 1
15.	Attaches oxygen	0 – 1
16.	Indicates need to continue chest compressions uninterrupted and to ventilate at a rate of approximately 10 breaths per minute	0 – 1
17.	Upon arrival of defibrillator, applies pads	0 – 1
18.	Assesses rhythm	0 – 1
19.	Attempts defibrillation	0 – 1
20.	Indicates need to continue resuscitation until resuscitation team arrives or until patient shows signs of life	0 – 1
21.	Total of candidate's checklist scores	
22.	Examiner's global score: CP, BP, BF, CF	
23.	Examiner's comments	

Appendix 6.2. Cannula Insertion and Intravenous Injection Skills Station

Candidate Instructions

SCENARIO: You are the HO on-call for Ward A3. Mrs Dacy Garcus is being managed for a gangrenous foot by another team. Her current medications include intravenous Ampiclox® which is to be administered now. You have been called to give the *iv* antibiotics.

YOUR TASK: Using the model arm provided, demonstrate to the examiner how you would go about this.

TIME ALLOWED: 10 minutes

PRACTICAL PROCEDURE STATION

Core Items on the Examiner's Rating Scale Would Include that the Candidate:

1. States intention to introduce self and confirm patient's name and date of birth or age
2. States intention to explain the need for intravenous antibiotics and the procedure, and to seek permission
3. States intention to check allergy status with patient and as documented on drug chart and patient's wristband
4. Checks vial of antibiotic for dose and expiry date
5. States that he would double-check drug name, dose and expiry with another member of medical or nursing staff
6. Refers to the *Hospital Formulary* (or other directory} for correct administration instructions
7. Washes hands and wears gloves
8. Applies tourniquet to model arm and selects a suitable vein
9. Cleans skin with an alcohol swab
10. Retracts skin to stabilize the vein and inserts cannula until flashback seen
11. Correctly advances cannula over needle, withdrawing needle partially to secure intravenous access
12. Releases tourniquet, completely withdraws the needle and caps the end of the cannula
13. Disposes of the needle safely
14. Secures cannula in place
15. Reconstitutes drug using correct volume of suitable diluent as per instructions
16. Draws reconstituted drug into syringe, administers via cannula at correct speed as per Formulary instructions
17. Disposes of drug ampoule safely
18. Signs and records time of administration on drug chart, asking the other health professional who checked the drugs to sign the chart as well
19. Examiner's global rating
20. Total of Candidate's checklist scores

Appendix 6.3. Oxygen Therapy Station

Candidate Instructions

SCENARIO: You are the duty registrar in A&E when Mr Dada Okoromu presents. He is 60 years old and was diagnosed of chronic obstructive airways disease about three years ago. He now presents complaining of increasing breathlessness at rest. He is in severe respiratory distress and needs oxygen.

YOUR TASK: Please administer the oxygen to him appropriately using the information, equipment, and materials provided, explaining to the examiner as you go along.

TIME ALLOWED: 10 minutes

Core Items on the Examiner's Rating Scale Would Include that the Candidate:

1. Introduces self and confirms patient's name and date of birth
2. Washes own hands.
3. Checks patient's oxygen saturation using pulse oximetry
4. Comments on adequacy of oxygen saturation
5. Offers arterial blood gas sampling
6. Correctly interprets blood gas results provided by the examiner
7. States need for oxygen therapy
8. Chooses a fixed-performance mask and valve to deliver 24 per cent oxygen
9. Correctly applies mask to patient, tightening the elastic straps and ensuring a good fit
10. Turns on oxygen at correct flow rate to deliver 24 percent
11. States intention to repeat arterial blood gas sampling after half an hour
12. Correctly interprets second blood gas results provided by the examiner
13. Changes concentration of oxygen appropriately
14. Prescribes oxygen on treatment chart
15. Examiner's global rating
16. Total of station's analytical scores
17. Total of candidate's analytical scores

Appendix 6.4. Death Confirmation Skill

PRACTICAL PROCEDURE STATION

Candidate Instructions

SCENARIO: You are the junior registrar doing the ward on-call. You have been phoned by the Ward Sister to confirm the death of a patient on the Geriatrics Ward.

YOUR TASK: Please demonstrate how you would confirm that the patient is dead using the mannequin provided, and explain your actions to the examiner as you go along. You may interact appropriately with the nurse in attendance. Document the certification.

TIME ALLOWED: 10 minutes

Core Items on the Examiner's Rating Scale Would Include that the Candidate:

1. Asks the nurse for a brief history of the background to the death
2. Confirms that the patient was not for resuscitation
3. States intention to read the patient's medical notes (You may be given a summary)
4. Confirms the identity of the 'patient'
5. Exposes the 'patient' adequately and observes, commenting on the absence of respiratory movements.
6. Palpates for a carotid pulse on both sides
7. Palpates for both radial pulses
8. Palpates for both femoral pulses
9. Auscultates over the praecordium for one minute, commenting on the absence of heart sounds
10. Auscultates over the chest for 3 minutes (or states intention to do so), commenting on the absence of breath sounds
11. Inspects the eyes with a pen torch for fixed and dilated pupils
12. Examines the fundi with an ophthalmoscope for segmentation of the retinal columns (or states intention to do so)
13. Washes hands
14. Writes the findings in the medical notes, stating the date and time of death (or states intention to do so)
15. Signs and prints name and designation in the medical notes (or states intention to do so)
16. States intention to direct the nurse as to what to do next

OSCE Skills for Trainees in Medicine

17. Examiner's global rating
18. Total of Station's analytical scores
19. Total of Candidate's analytical scores

NB: A death is documented in the medical notes in the following form or some modification of same.

The Death Certificate Document should:
1. State date and time assessment started.
2. State whom you are: e.g. JR on Ward Call
3. State: Asked to confirm death by nursing staff. Medical notes reviewed and noted that either patient was not for resuscitation and for supportive care only, with imminent death expected or for resuscitation and efforts you made.
   - No cardiovascular effort.
   - No respiratory effort.
   - Pupils fixed and dilated.
   - Segmentation of retinal columns on fundoscopic examination.
4. State Date and time death certified: dd/mm/yyyy; hh, mm Rest in peace
5. Dr's Name, Designation, contact (Phone or Bleep), Signature. Date

Appendix 6.5. Blood Transfusion Skills

Candidate Instructions

SCENARIO: You are the HO with the Registrar on-call. Dr Silver Pam is a 75-year-old man with a known history of peptic ulcer disease. He presents with melena and haematemesis. His supine BP is 100/60 mmHg, and his PCV 14%. The registrar after review has obtained blood to be transfused.

YOUR TASK: To administer Mr. Pam's first unit of blood. Please demonstrate how you would do this using the model arm provided.

TIME ALLOWED: 10 minutes

Core Items on the Examiner's Rating Scale Would Include that the Candidate:

PRACTICAL PROCEDURE STATION

1. States intention to introduce self and confirm patient's name and date of birth
2. States intention to explain the need for a blood transfusion and the procedure, and to seek the patient's permission
3. Ensures that baseline observations have been recorded
4. Washes hands and wears gloves
5. Applies tourniquet to model arm and selects a suitable vein
6. Cleans skin with an alcohol wipe
7. Retracts skin to stabilize the vein and inserts appropriate sized cannula until flashback seen
8. Correctly advances cannula over needle, withdrawing needle partially to secure intravenous access
9. Releases tourniquet, completely withdraws the needle and caps the end of the cannula
10. Disposes of the needle safely
11. Secures cannula in place
12. Chooses correct *i.v.* administration set and primes with normal saline
13. Runs normal saline through the cannula
14. Checks the patient's hospital number, name, date of birth and blood group as labelled on the unit of blood against the accompanying sheet from the blood bank with a qualified health professional (nurse/doctor)
15. Checks the hospital number, date of birth and name as labelled on the unit of blood with the patient's wristband, and states intention to check also with the patient himself
16. Documents the serial number of the unit of blood on the medicine chart and signs it, asking the other health professional who checked the blood to sign the chart as well
17. Correctly changes the bag of saline to blood
18. Commences the blood infusion at the rate prescribed on the chart
19. Ensures that appropriate observations for adverse reactions will be commenced by the nursing staff
20. Examiner's global rating
21. Total of station's analytical scores
22. Total of candidate's analytical scores

Appendix 6.6 General Basic Life Support Algorithm

1. Check for movement and/or responsiveness.
2. If not moving and/or responsive, call emergency number and get Automated External Defibrillator (AED) if available.
3. Open airway and check breathing.
4. If not breathing, give two breaths.
5. If no change after giving two breaths, check pulse.
5A. If there is a pulse, give one breath every five to six seconds, and recheck pulse every two minutes.
6. If no pulse, give 30 compressions (hard and fast @ 100/min with little or no interruptions) and two breaths until AED gets there, (Advanced Life Support (ALS) arrives, and/or patient starts to move.

WHEN AN AED/DEFIBRILLATOR ARRIVES.

7. Check heart rhythm.
8. If shockable, give one shock and resume CPR for five cycles.
9. If not shockable, resume CPR for five cycles. Check rhythm every five cycles (i.e. about every two minutes), and continue CPR until ALS arrives or patient starts to move.

Appendix 6.7. American Heart Association (AHA) Basic Life Support Algorithm

Adult basic life support sequence

1. Make sure the victim, any bystander, and you are safe.
2. Check the victim for a response:
   Gently shake his shoulders and ask loudly, 'Are you all right?'

3A. *If he responds:*
- Leave him in the position in which you find him provided there is no further danger.
- Try to find out what is wrong with him and get help if needed.
- Reassess him regularly.

3B. *If he does not respond:*
- Shout for help.
- Turn the victim onto his back and then open the airway using head tilt and chin lift:
  o Place your hand on his forehead and gently tilt his head back.

- o   With your fingertips under the point of the victim's chin, lift the chin to open the airway.

4. Keeping the airway open, (look, listen, and feel for normal breathing).
- Look for chest movement.
- Listen at the victim's mouth for breath sounds.
- Feel for air on your cheek.
- Look, listen, and feel for no more than 10 s to determine if the victim is breathing normally.
- If you have any doubt whether breathing is normal, act as if it is not normal.

5A. *If he is breathing normally:*
- Turn him into the recovery position.
- Summon help from the ambulance service by mobile phone. If this is not possible, send a bystander. Leave the victim only if no other way of obtaining help is possible.
- Continue to assess that breathing remains normal.
- If there is any doubt about the presence of normal breathing, start CPR (5B).

5B. *If he is not breathing normally:*
- Ask someone to call for an ambulance and bring an AED if available. If you are on your own, use your phone to call for an ambulance. Leave the victim *only when* no other option exists for getting help.
- Start chest compression as follows:
  - o   Kneel by the side of the victim.
  - o   Place the heel of one hand in the centre of the victim's chest (the lower half of the victim's sternum).
  - o   Place the heel of your other hand on top of the first hand.
  - o   Interlock the fingers of your hands and ensure that pressure is not applied over the victim's ribs. Do not apply any pressure over the upper abdomen or the bottom end of the sternum.
  - o   Position yourself vertically above the victim's chest and, with your arms straight, press down on the sternum 5 - 6 cm.
  - o   After each compression, release all the pressure on the chest without losing contact between your hands and the sternum.

o   Repeat at a rate of 100 – 120 per minute. Compression and release should take an equal amount of time.

6A. Combine chest compression with rescue breaths:

- After 30 compressions open the airway again using head tilt and chin lift.
- Pinch the soft part of the victim's nose closed, using the index finger and thumb of your hand on his forehead.
- Allow his mouth to open, but maintain chin lift.
- Take a normal breath and place your lips around his mouth, making sure that you have a good seal.
- Blow steadily into his mouth whilst watching for his chest to rise; take about one second to make his chest rise as in normal breathing; this is an effective rescue breath.
- Maintaining head tilt and chin lift, take your mouth away from the victim and watch for his chest to fall as air comes out.
- Take another normal breath and blow into the victim's mouth once more to give a total of two effective rescue breaths. The two breaths should not take more than 5 s. Then return your hands without delay to the correct position on the sternum and give a further 30 chest compressions.
- Continue with chest compressions and rescue breaths in a ratio of 30:2.
- Stop to recheck the victim only if he starts to show signs of regaining consciousness, such as coughing, opening his eyes, speaking, or moving purposefully AND starts to breathe normally; otherwise **do not interrupt resuscitation.**
- If the initial rescue breath of each sequence does not make the chest rise as in normal breathing, then, before your next attempt:
    o   Check the victim's mouth and remove any visible obstruction.
    o   Recheck that there is adequate head tilt and chin lift.
- Do not attempt more than two breaths each time before returning to chest compressions. If there is more than one rescuer present, another should take over CPR about every 1-2 min to prevent fatigue. Ensure the minimum of delay during the changeover of rescuers, and do not interrupt chest compressions.

6B. Compression-only CPR

- If you are *not trained* to, or are unwilling to give rescue breaths, *give chest compressions only.*
- If chest compressions only are given, these should be continuous at a rate of 100 - 120 min^{-1}.
- Stop to recheck the victim only if he starts to show signs of regaining consciousness, such as coughing, opening his eyes, speaking, or moving purposefully AND starts to breathe normally; otherwise **do not interrupt resuscitation.**

7. *Continue resuscitation until:*

- qualified help arrives and takes over,
- **or** the victim starts to show signs of regaining consciousness, such as coughing, opening his eyes, speaking, or moving purposefully AND starts to breathe normally, **OR** you become exhausted.

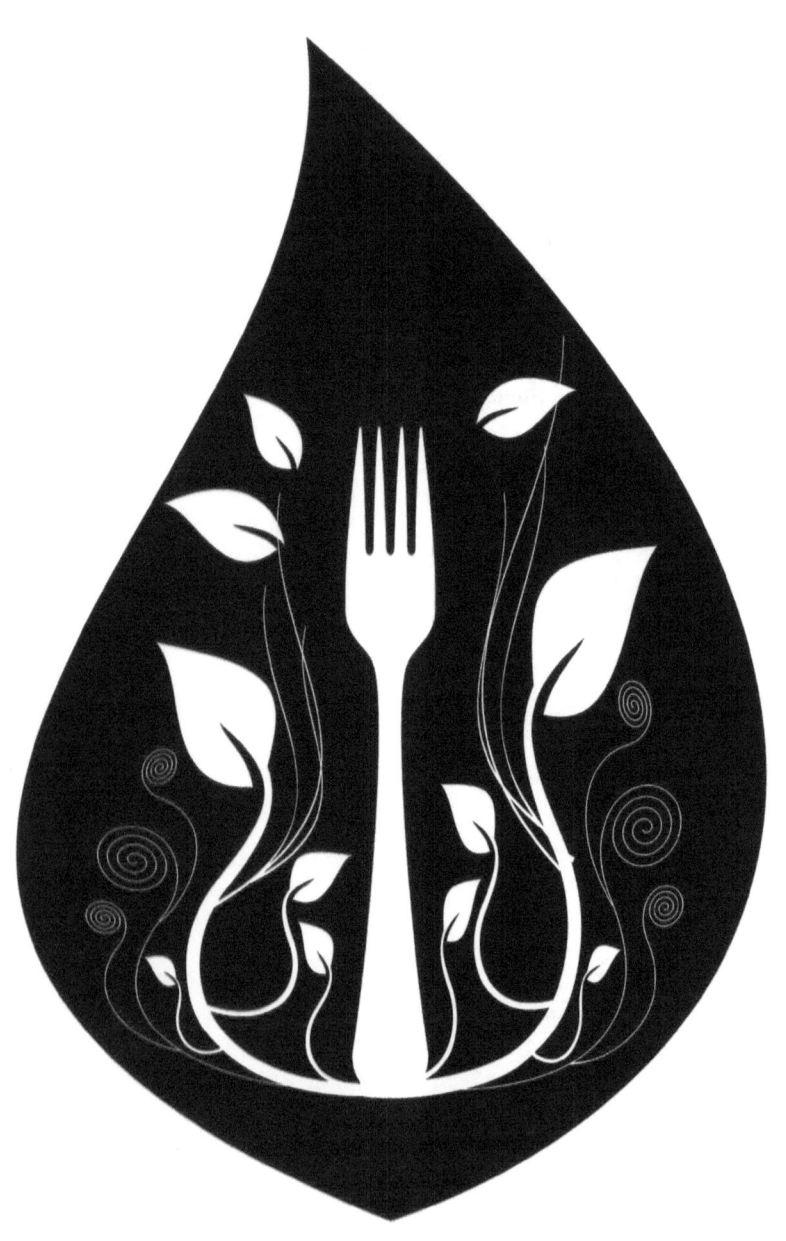

7

Objective Structured Practical Examination

7.1. Introduction

7.2. Purpose and Types of OSPE stations

7.3. Objective Structured Practical Examination Circuit

7.4. Features of an OSPE Circuit

7.5. Assessing Candidate Performance in OSPE

7.6. Hints and Tips for the OSPE Candidate

7.7 Examples of OSPE Stations

7.8. Chapter Seven Summary

7.9. Chapter Seven Recap Exercises

7.10. Bibliography and Resources

7.11. Appendix: Some Plausible Themes for OSPE Stations

7.1. INTRODUCTION

Objective **S**tructured **P**ractical **E**xamination (OSPE), one of the variants of OSCE, is particularly applicable where patient encounter is not much needed. It is widely used in the assessment of students in both clinical and basic medical sciences. The reasons that necessitated the introduction of OSCE in the clinical sciences also informed the birth of OSPE, especially in the basic medical sciences, the pathological sciences, and in some aspects of the clinical sciences in medicine and allied professions. Most of what is said about OSCE (including structure and process) equally applies to OSPE. Variations in experiments selected and inter-examiner gradings of candidate's competencies are issues students and examination organizers would want minimized. The only variable in a student assessment exercise should be the candidate's performance, and not any other confounding or lurking factors. The OSPE serves to help to obviate the shortcomings inherent in the traditional assessment of practical skills.

In an OSPE exercise students are tested on various cognitive and psychomotor skills such as: clinical scenario, identification and interpretation of histological slides or micrographs, anatomical or pathological specimens, photographs, X-rays, and CT-scans. Laboratory and clinical reports can also be used. Tasks may include asking candidates to calculate, draw, label or interpret a diagram or a graph.

7.2. PURPOSE AND TYPES OF OSPE STATIONS

The main purpose of an OSPE exercise is to test the basic practical skills of trainees. OSPE harnesses the versatility of the OSCE approach in assessment to overcome the disadvantages of testing practical skills in the traditional way. The emphasis in OSPE is on assessment of practical abilities while the candidate is directly observed as they perform the task rather than just testing theoretical knowledge. OSPE, like OSCE, has the advantage of being able to cover a large area of the curriculum and of being able to *treat* all candidates in a similar manner.

POTENTIAL USES OF OSPE

Objective **S**tructured **P**ractical **E**xamination, like OSCE, can be employed formatively and summatively in the basic medical sciences (of physiology, pharmacology, biochemistry, and anatomy) and in the pathological sciences (of microbiology, chemical pathology, histopathology, and haematology). Core clinical areas in medicine and allied health professions may also find it useful to incorporate OSPE-type stations into their OSCEs.

SKILLS EXAMINABLE IN OSPE

Several practical and related skills can be examined in an OSPE exercise. Such OSPE-assessable competencies include but not limited to the following:

Analysing results of experiment	Planning an experiment
Applying knowledge and evidence	Simulated skills
	Special tasks
Laboratory based measurement	Using an equipment: e.g. ECG machine, Glucometer
Laboratory procedures	
Making decisions/problem solving	X-ray, laboratory preps and results
Microscopy skills	

Stations in an OSPE may be classified on the basis of competency being assessed and/or the presence of an examiner at the station. However, you will most likely meet four types of OSPE station besides rest stations: general scientific experiment station, basic clinical skills station, data interpretation station, and a *viva voce* station.

Objective **S**tructured **P**ractical **E**xamination encounters may also be divided into *procedure stations (practical or clinical) and response stations*. As in OSCE, a procedure station is manned or observed. A response or an unmanned station may be related to the previous station (*couplet station*) or be a totally new scenario. Most of the types of stations used in OSCE such as structured oral examination and written exercises may also be found in OSPE. In a science experiment station, candidates may be asked to identify equipment parts, assemble equipment, go through an experiment procedure, and make observations. They may also be asked to interpret resultant data from which they can draw conclusions. However, interpreting resultant data and drawing conclusions may be left to a succeeding *couplet station*.

Clinical stations in OSPE are similar to those in OSCE (such as history taking, physical examination or a clinical procedures, interpretation of lab results, and communication etc). The clinical stations in OSPE are however usually at a lower level of clinical competence than in the OSCE for clinical students.

7.3. OBJECTIVE STRUCTURED PRACTICAL EXAMINATION CIRCUIT

As mentioned earlier, stations in OSPE often include general scientific experiment station, basic clinical skills station, data interpretation station, and practical procedures. The collection of the tasks for a particular examination exercise is referred to as an *OSPE circuit*. The number of stations in an OSPE circuit generally varies from 10 – 20 stations but may be fewer in formative assessment exercises or more in postgraduate examinations. Each station lasts 3-5 minutes. A schematic representation of an OSPE circuit is shown in Figure 7.1.

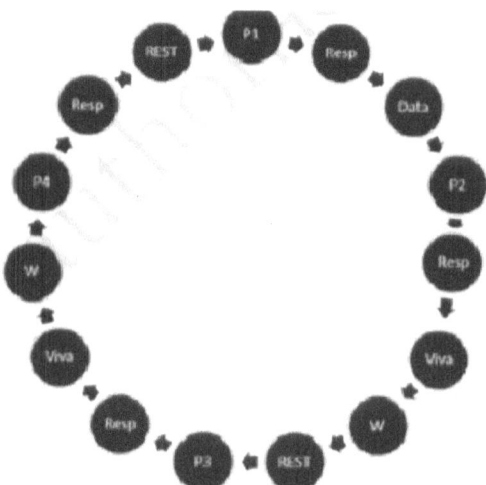

Figure 7. 1. A Schema of an OSPE Circuit. *Note the similarity in structure of OSPE to an OSCE circuit. P stands for a procedure or manned station, W for a written or unmanned station, R for a response or couplet station being dependent on the preceding station. The unmanned independent or written stations can be pulled and examined at a different location as projected slides, printed booklets, or a steeple chase. A rest station occurs after every eight or so stations.*

7.4. FEATURES OF AN OSPE CIRCUIT

In an OSPE circuit, some stations will have examiners (and sometimes an SP) present. Like at OSCE stations, your instruction materials will include a description of a problem or clinical scenario and then instructions telling you what your task is at the station. The OSPE procedure is very similar to that of an OSCE. If you are unfamiliar with OSCE, you should read (or read again) Chapter 2 on an overview of the OSCE system of assessment. Table 7.1 shows the main elements to be found at an OSPE station.

Table 7.1. Features of OSPE Stations

	Station element	*Comment*
1	Station Number	Provided for all stations
2	Station Title	Provided for all stations
3	Station Construct or Purpose	Provided for all stations
4	Time Allowed	Provided for all stations
5	Scenario or Stem to Question	Problem solving
6	Candidate Instructions	Provided for all stations
7	Technician Instructions	Tasks on experiments or needing equipment.
8	Instructions for Simulated Patients	Stations with SPs
9	Questions, Marksheet and Schedule	For written stations
10	Charts, Graphs or Diagrams	Especially for written stations
11	Specimens	Manned or unmanned
12	Checklist or Rating Scale	Manned /procedure stations
13	Feedback Forms	For entire OSPE or station

Staff at an OSPE Station

At a manned OSPE station, there will always be an examiner or rater who may be a teacher or some other persons with technical expertise. There may also be a simulated patient or an actor at stations assessing elementary technical skills. Where there is need to manipulate an instrument or device, a laboratory person will also be available to guide you. Some stations have a local time keeper to help you manage your time well. Unmanned stations have no examiners or SPs present but assistants or laboratory personnel may be available to assist or guide you.

Information Elements at an OSPE Station

General Information about Station

STATION NUMBER: this is the circuit identity number.

STATION TITLE refers to the competency being tested e.g. microscopy.

STATION CONSTRUCT states the purpose of the station and may read something like: The purpose of this station is to test the candidate's ability to ... (set up experiment, identify abnormality, use a specified equipment etc.).

TIME ALLOWED is usually about 3 to 5 minutes for the task to be completed; after which the candidate then moves to the next station.

STEM OR SCENARIO: This is introductory information on the task to be performed, e.g. patient complaining of painful urination.

Information and Instructions for the Candidate

The section featuring information for the candidate is the most relevant aspect to you, the candidate. It has several parts:

SCENARIO OR SETTING: This states whom the candidate is (e.g. what level) and the setting of the problem. E.g., You are the pathology registrar at the lab and to whom this CSF from a child with acute fever is sent.

YOUR TASK: Describes what you are expected to do e.g. *To examine and report on the CSF slide from this patient.*

TIME ALLOWED: States how much time you have to stay at the station; the time includes any time for interaction with the examiners if this is required. Programme yourself to work within the time allocated.

ADDITIONAL INFORMATION: Further instruction may be given such as... examiners will ask you questions, you may write notes, information will be used at the next station, etc.

Information for Laboratory Staff and Simulated Patient

Appropriate instructions are given to the laboratory staff and/or simulated patients when a station involves such persons.

Materials and Equipment at OSPE Stations

Invariably, for an OSPE, there will be stations with materials and equipment for experiments or other tasks. You should therefore be familiar with such things as weighing scales, colorimeters, sphygmomanometers, microscope and others (Fig 7.2) required to perform the common procedures listed in Appendix 7.1

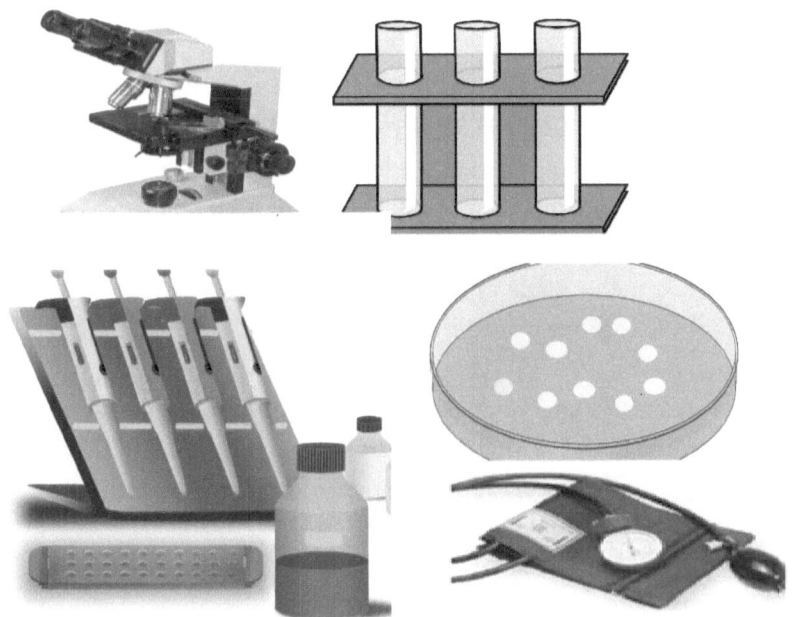

Figure 7.2. Potential Test Materials at OSPE Stations. *The test material at an OSPE station is dictated by the prescribed task to be performed and will usually include equipment and devices for common procedures and experiments. All the aspects of an experiment from planning through setting it up to interpretation of results can feature at an OSPE station. In addition viva and simple practical skills assessment may also be found in an OSPE.*

7.5. ASSESSING CANDIDATE PERFORMANCE IN OSPE

Your performance outcome in the entire OSPE is the aggregate of your performances at all the circuit stations. Scoring a candidate's performance at an individual OSPE station can take the form of one or more of the following: *checklist, rating scale, use of marking scheme, and global rating*. Checklists, rating scales, and global rating scales are used for manned stations while model answers with marking schemes are used for static or written stations.

The task at a manned or interactive station in OSPE is broken down into its constituent parts. Appropriate marks are awarded to each sub-task, using a structured predetermined checklist or rating scale as in OSCE. Static or Written Stations which are also referred to as *unobserved or unmanned stations* (see Chapter 8 on the *Written Station*) have no examiners physically present at the location. A static station consists of information about a patient, experiment, equipment or some other theme about which questions are posed for the candidate to answer in a written form. The format consists of a scenario or stem, followed by questions to be answered.

7.6. HINTS AND TIPS FOR THE OSPE CANDIDATE

The suggestions and advice made in Chapters 2 and 6 on how to improve student performance in OSCE are equally germane to the OSPE candidate. The OSPE candidate is enjoined to read same along with the additional comments made here.

The OSPE requires you to have good grasp of such practical skills as common experiments CPR, urine testing, microscopy etc. Learn how to recognise structures and be able to describe things clearly and concisely. Stay within the limits of the examination. You also need to be good in communicating with your examiners and/or simulated patients.

7. 7. EXAMPLES OF OSPE STATIONS

7.7.1. An Observed or Manned OSPE Station: Biochemical Analysis

Instructions to the candidate

> STEM: This is a solution of glucose, labelled G.
> YOUR TASK: Analyse the sample of glucose solution labelled G using the spectrophotometer provided. Do a running commentary, telling the examiner what you are doing and/or why.
> TIME ALLOWED: Five minutes

Scoring Instructions to the Examiner

Please rate the performance of the candidate using the scheme/checklist (Table 7.2) provided. The Table shows the type of major steps that would be listed for award of marks by the examiner at a station like this.

Table 7. 2. Scoring an Experiment Station: Analytic Determination

	Procedure Activity	Rating (marks)		
		Adequate	Inadequate	Not done
1	Checks and confirms that all materials required for the analysis are present	1	0	0
2	Adjusts the spectrophotometer to the right wavelength (at 530 nm for glucose)	2	1	0
3	Measures and adds 1 ml of reagent blank into the cuvette	2	1	0
4	Places the cuvette in the cuvette holder and closes same	0.5	0	0
5	Adjusts zero absorbance for the reagent blank	2	1	0
6	Empties and dries cuvette	1	0	0
7	Adds right amount (1ml) of sample into the cuvette and measures the absorbance	2	1	0
8	Answer to Question: How will you calculate the concentration of glucose in solution G from your reading?	3	1	0
9	Checklist total			
10	Global rating of performance: CP BP BF CF			

BF, borderline fail; BP, borderline pass; CF, clear fail; CP, clear pass.

7.7.2. An Unmanned OSPE Station: Microscopy

Candidate Instruction

SCENARIO: A woman who complains of abdominal swelling had surgery. The slide under the microscope is the histology of a biopsy of an abdominal organ from the operation.

YOUR TASK: Answer the following questions based on your microscopic findings.

TIME ALLOWED: Five minutes

Questions

QUESTION 1. What organ is this? (Maximum score, 4 marks)
QUESTION 2. List the two main abnormalities present on the slide. (2 marks each)
QUESTION 3. What is the most likely aetiology of this lesion? (2 marks)

Model answers

Model answers are for the use of the examiners who have been asked to grade the candidates' answers. The most correct answer attracts maximum marks while plausible but less correct answers attract lower marks. Hypothetical answers to the questions could be as follows:

ANSWER TO QUESTION 1: *What organ is this? (4 marks).*
Liver, 4 marks; Other, 0-2 marks.

ANSWER TO QUESTION 2. *List the two main abnormalities present in this slide? (2 marks each)*
- Fibrosis (2 marks)
- Nodular regeneration (2 marks)
- Nodules (1 mark)
- Other, 0

ANSWER TO QUESTION 3. *What is the most likely aetiology of this lesion? (2 marks)*
- Chronic hepatitis B infection (2 marks)
- Hepatitis (1 mark)
- Chronic alcoholism (0.5 mark)
- Other accepted cause of cirrhosis (0.5 mark)
- Totally wrong answers (0 mark)

MAXIMUM TOTAL SCORE: 10 marks
CANDIDATE'S TOTAL SCORE: (Sum up)

7.7.3. OSPE Station: Clinical Measurement

Information about the Station

STATION CONSTRUCT: The purpose of this station is to test the candidate's ability to take a blood pressure accurately.
TIME ALLOWED: 5 minutes
SCENARIO: James Daudu is a 19-year-old man who has come for a pre-admission medical assessment.

STRUCTURED PRACTICAL EXAMINATION

Candidate Instructions

SCENARIO: Mr James Daudu a 19-year-old man has a letter offering him admission to study medicine at a top university. He needs a medical certificate of fitness including a report on his blood pressure.

YOUR TASK. You are the University Medical Officer to whom James comes at the Health Centre for the pre-admission medical assessment.
   a. Please measure his blood pressure.
   b. You should tell the examiner what you are doing and why.
   c. Please discuss your findings with James.
   d. The examiners will ask you some questions.

TIME ALLOWED: You have 5 minutes for this task.

Instructions to Simulated Patient

You are a 19-year-old man about to enter the University. As part of your pre-admission requirements you have come for a blood pressure check. Discuss the blood pressure with the doctor as you were previously briefed. Do not remind or prompt any candidate if they fail to perform any aspect of the procedure.

Instruction to the Station Examiner on Scoring BP Measurement

CHECKLIST RATING. Using the checklist provided (Table 7.3). Please rate the performance of the candidate on each component item as: *Done well (1 mark), poorly done or not done (0 mark)*

GLOBAL RATING: In addition to rating individual task components, please globally grade the overall performance of the candidate. The global rating should be independent of your checklist scores of the candidate's performance at this station.

Table 7.3. A Checklist for Measuring Blood Pressure

	Task component objective	Done well	Poorly/ not done
1	Initial approach: Establishes rapport and makes the patient at ease	1	0
2	Washes hands before and after procedure	1	0
3	Selects/comments on appropriate sphyg cuff size	2	0
4	Positions patient and equipment appropriately.	1	0
5	Exposes the arms, removes any restrictions, supports arm at heart level	1	0
6	Ensures that the Hg manometer is upright and at his/her eye level	1	0
7	Palpates the brachial artery; wraps cuff smoothly and snugly around arm	1	0
8	Inflates the cuff, determines rough SBP by palpating the artery	1	0
9	Inflates cuff fully, applies stethoscope, and re-inflates to 20 – 30 mmHg above palpated SBP.	2	0
10	Deflates cuff slowly until SBP and DBP recorded while listening	1	0
11	Deflates fully after each reading	1	0
12	Repeats (or requests to repeat) BP in same position after at least 2 min	1	0
13	Removes sphyg, folds and replaces in container.	1	0
14	Tells, or hands over to the patient the written readings, followed by a brief discussion of the readings	2	0
15	Thanks the patient	1	0
17	Answer to Examiner: What was the BP?	2	0
18	Total checklist score for station		
19	Total checklist score for candidate		
20	Global rating: Very good; Good; Borderline; Clear fail		
21	General Comments on candidate or station		

BP, blood pressure; DBP, diastolic blood pressure; SBP, systolic blood pressure; Sphyg, Sphygmomanometer

STRUCTURED PRACTICAL EXAMINATION

7.7.4. Pharmacy Task Station

Candidate Instructions

SETTING: You are a pharmacy intern who has been provided with prepared benzyl benzoate emulsion.

YOUR TASK: Dispense 20 ml of the emulsion to Jaro Korotu, a 15-year-old boy with scabies. His ID number is 72516

TIME ALLOWED: 5 minutes

Examiner Instructions

Please score the candidate's performance for each listed item as follows:
- Satisfactorily done: 2 marks
- Done but Unsatisfactorily: 1 mark
- Not done: 0

Please enter your awarded score:
1. Measures 20 ml correctly: ....
2. Puts the measured vol into a dark bottle: ....
3. Puts a cork on it: ....
4. Puts a dark coloured cap over it: ....
5. Ties a pharmaceutical knot: ....
6. Puts primary labels:
    a. The emulsion ....
    b. Patient's Name ....
    c. Patient's Age ....
    d. Patient's Sex ....
    e. Patient's ID Number ....
7. Written Directions
    a. Apply all over the body from neck, downwards, after a thorough cleansing bath ....
    b. Repeat the application after 12 h, ...
    c. Followed by a change of clothing after 24h ....
8. Secondary labels
    a. For external use only ....
    b. Shake the bottle before use ....
9. Intern Pharmacist's information
    a. Name-------------------------------------

    b. Signature ---------------------------------
    c. Date--
    d. Address ------------------------------------
    e. Registration Number ----------------------
10. 10. General: Neatly dispensed. ....
11. 11. MAXIMUM TOTAL SCORE: X marks ....
12. CANDIDATE'S TOTAL SCORE: (Add up) ....

7.8. CHAPTER SEVEN SUMMARY

- **O**bjective **S**tructured **P**ractical **E**xamination (OSPE) is a multiple station examination similar to OSCE where candidates rotate through a series of encounters referred to as *stations*.
- At each OSPE station, candidates have to perform a standardised task.
- All candidates perform the same tasks and are graded in the same structured manner
- Grading performance in OSPE consists of direct observations using checklists and rating scales as well as short answer questions or multiple choice questions
- OSPE is mainly used for the preclinical and pathological courses but can also be used in assessing some aspects of clinical medicine.
- The OSPE is a much fairer assessment than traditional practical examinations. Its advantages far outweigh its shortcomings.

The following are some of the key features of OSPE:
- ***Similarities to OSCE***
    o Structured
    o Multiple station delivery
    o Variety of skills and tasks
    o Several observers or raters needed for every candidate
    o All candidates take same test
    o Structured scoring of performance of candidate
    o Fairer exams than traditional methods
- ***Advantages of OSPE***
    o Reduces bias

- Uniform level of assessment
- Large number of skills can be assessed within relatively short time
- Wider sampling of curriculum content
- Tool has a high reliability
- Tailor-made assessment of skills as per importance
- Highly objective in grading due to structuring
- Recall bias minimised
- Less duplication of equipment
- Less preparation for each task
- Overall reduced cost
- Supervision is easier

- **Disadvantages of OSPE**
  - Standard time duration for all tests, difficult to increase or decrease
  - Requires serious planning
  - Requires validation
  - Requires high degree of team work
  - Tasks broken down for ease of assessment, smacks of artificiality
  - Security threats due to so many people being involved

7.9. CHAPTER SEVEN RECAP EXERCISES

1. List four types of stations that may be found in an OSPE run.
2. List five assessable skills in an OSPE in your discipline.
3. At what type of OSPE stations would the following scoring modes be used in OSPE?
   a. Checklist
   b. Rating scale
   c. Model answers
4. Think of an OSPE circuit in your specialty that consists of 16 stations. List tasks for stations like performing an experiment, interpretation of result data, *viva voce*, written (unmanned problems), calculations, labelling etc. to constitute the circuit. Provide for two rest stations and ensure that the tasks are doable in 3 minutes.

7.10. BIBLIOGRAPHY AND RESOURCES. See page 249

7.11. APPENDICES

Appendix 7.1. Some Plausible Themes for OSPE Stations
1. Cardiopulmonary resuscitation (CPR)
2. Detection of bleeding time and clotting time
3. Detection of lung volumes and capacities (spirometry)
4. Determination of blood groups (both ABO and/or Rh)
5. Determination of erythrocyte sedimentation rate (ESR)
6. Determination of platelet count
7. Determination of red blood cell count
8. Determination of red cell indices and haematocrit
9. Determination of white blood cell count
10. Effect of exercise and posture on blood pressure
11. Electrocardiography (recording of ECG)
12. Estimation of haemoglobin
13. Examination of arterial pulse, jugular venous pulse
14. Identification of heart sounds
15. Measurement of blood pressure at rest
16. Microscopy: preparation of slide and focusing
17. Mounting a compound microscope
18. R.B.C Fragility test
19. Recording of chest movement by stethography
20. Temperature recording at rest and immediately after exercise

8

Written or Static Station

8.1. Introduction

8.2. Purpose and Formats of a Written Station

8.3. Competencies Assessable at a Written Station

8.4. Elements at a Written Station

8.5. Advice to the Candidate about Written Stations

8.6. Illustrative Examples of a Written Station

8.7. Chapter Eight Summary

8.8. Chapter Eight Recap Exercises

8.9. Bibliography and Resources

8.1. INTRODUCTION

The principal active stations in an OSCE circuit are the: clinical stations (with patients and examiners present); practical stations with examiners present ± patients (see Chapter 6), structured *viva voce* stations with examiners ± equipment or data (see Chapter 9), and unmanned stations. The unmanned station is also variously referred to as static, non-interactive, written, post-encounter probe or question station. Written stations are similar to so-called practicals or data interpretation of some institutions and may feature in both OSCE and OSPE.

Written stations are encounters that usually do not require the presence of patients or examiners. Candidates, therefore, do not have any physical interaction with patients or examiners at such a station but examination assistants may be present. Written stations which are related to previous stations may be post-encounter, probe or couplet stations. Early in the development of OSCE, written stations were mainly question stations based on the preceding performance stations. In current practice, these written stations can stand alone or be coupled to another station. Un-manned stations can be included in an OSCE to examine other skills and competencies related to patient care and management.

8.2. PURPOSE AND FORMATS OF WRITTEN STATIONS

Written stations serve several purposes in an OSCE or OSPE. When incorporated into an OSCE/OSPE, written stations help to increase the number of stations, thereby enhancing the reliability of the exercise. When there is a shortage of examiners, some of the interactive stations can be converted to un-manned ones. Written stations may be used in place of so-called practical examinations or data interpretations in some examination systems.

The structure of a static station consists of a problem created from a clinical scenario or other matter being presented to the candidate. A static task involves responding in writing to a set of structured questions based on the information provided. Question formats on the theme may be in the form of short answer questions, labelling diagrams, or providing answers to questions in MCQ formats. Written unmanned stations may be included in the OSCE or OSPE circuit or may be administered separately at another time and location.

8.3. COMPETENCIES ASSESSABLE AT A WRITTEN STATION

Several competencies can be assessed at a written OSCE station. Such competencies vary from partly simple recall tasks to assessment of attitudes. Written-examinable competencies in OSCE include:

- Basic and clinical science knowledge
- Clinical reasoning
- Death certification
- Decision making
- Ethics and medico-legal knowledge
- Health promotion and disease
- prevention
- Judgement
- Patient investigation
- Patient management
- Personal development
- Prescription writing

A variation of the un-manned station is where the candidate interacts with the patient, takes notes and moves to the next station to interact with the examiners, the emphasis here may be on record keeping. Alternatively, the students' notes can be graded on their own.

8.4. ELEMENTS A WRITTEN STATION

Staff at a Written Station.

As mentioned earlier, at an un-manned or written station you will not meet an examiner or a patient. There might, however, be an assistant or a technician to assist you when the need arises or as instructed.

Information Elements at a Written Station

At a written station, you will be presented with information describing a problem, patient scenario or image along with questions related to the problem or data. A description of the station with its elements such as station title, construct, competency, and domain to be assessed would be provided as well as instructions to the candidate and the examiner who would grade the answer scripts later.

OSCE Skills for Trainees in Medicine

Test Materials at a Written Station

Task questions at written stations can be based a number of sources. The most popular of these sources are patient laboratory results, imaging (X-rays, CTs, MRIs, and ultrasonographic prints) and clinical pictures. Questions can also be based on instruments, see Figures 8.1 and 8.2.

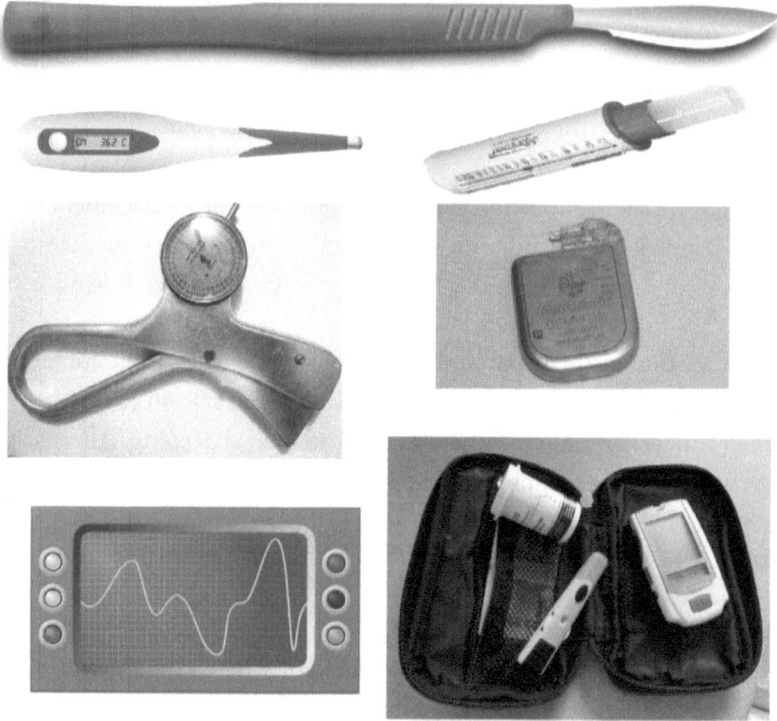

Figure 8.1 Instruments and Devices that May Be Found an OSCE Written Station. *Common tasks on such materials include identification, labelling, indications for use, precautions and other questions related to practical use. What about identifying the instruments and devices shown?*

STATIC STATION

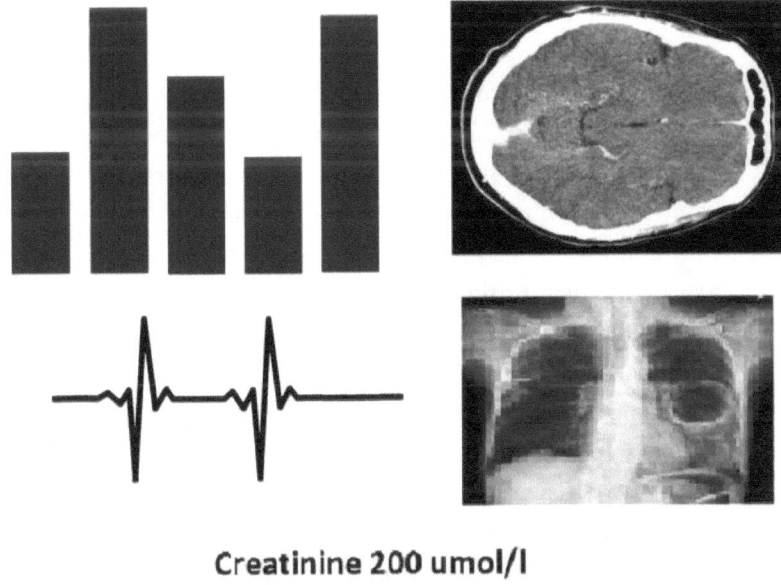

Creatinine 200 umol/l
Urea   4 mol/l
Na   140 mmol/l
Potassium 2.6 mol/l
Bicarbonate 34 mmol/l

Figure 8.2. Images and Other Test Materials that Might be at Written Stations. *Such materials may also be found at an oral examination station.*

8.5. ADVICE TO THE CANDIDATE ABOUT WRITTEN STATIONS

Passing or failing the written or un-manned stations may depend on a number of factors. If your knowledge of the topics is inadequate in a few stations, you can still pass the entire examination as most examining authorities do not include *veto stations* whereby a poor performance at a particular station can spell doom. Rather it is your average performance across all stations (manned and written) that determines your fate. The following information and measures can help improve your performance at the written stations of the OSCE/OSPE:

1. The questions at a written station may be in the form of MCQs, labelling, or short answers questions. Your response should therefore be appropriate.

2. As always, carefully read the instructions and the problem before answering.
3. If you are required to write down the answers, do so legibly.
4. Some questions and/or answers may be awarded higher marks than others, depending on their adjudged importance.
5. In answering questions, follow the instructions very closely. A common mistake is for candidates to provide more than what is required. Thus if asked of two important abnormalities present on a film, some candidates would write three or four. Lenient examination systems may score only the first two and ignore the rest; some other systems would score the candidate zero for failing to follow instructions. Small things matter!
6. When two answers are correct but one more so than the other, the more correct answer would attract a higher score. Therefore, always provide your answers in decreasing order of importance or accuracy. Thus if asked what is the most likely aetiological agent causing tetanus in a patient, if one candidate writes *Clostridium* and another says *Clostridium tetani*, the latter answer should carry higher marks for being more specific. So be thorough!
7. It sounds unbelievable, yet some candidates fail to write or affix their IDs on the answer scripts.
8. Avoid the temptation to keep altering your answers, especially where you are carrying the answer booklets around the circuit.
9. Be clear of the differences among common terms like *list, outline, short answers and others frequently used in* in written stations. See the glossary for some definitions of common terms.
10. If you are told to list or give a certain number of answers, write and number them.
11. The question sheet is for all the candidates in the circuit. Do not take it away, write on it, or deface it in any way. It can be annoying and/or frustrating to co-examinees if this happens.
12. Stationery (pencils, pens, erasers etc.) may be provided. But having your own to use if allowed is better.
13. Practise generously on past or similar questions.

8.6. ILLUSTRATIVE EXAMPLES OF WRITTEN STATION

Note that the format of the written station is generally similar to other stations in OSCE, as they consist of a problem or scenario followed by questions to which to react appropriately. The required response is however different to the task at a manned station. The station may consist of the usual general elements of station identification, purpose, problem or scenario and clear instructions to the candidate as in the example shown below or some of the elements may be omitted.

8.6.1. Station X: Written Station Based on Investigation Results

General Information about Station X
STATION NUMBER: **X**
STATION TITLE: Written Station
STATION CONSTRUCT OR PURPOSE. To test the ability of the candidate to make an X-ray diagnosis and initiate further management.

Briefing and Instructions to Candidate
> STATION CONSTRUCT: To test your ability to make an X-ray diagnosis and initiate further management.
> SCENARIO. You are the registrar in A&E when the patient described below presents.

Mr Yobu Tinka, a 23 - year-old undergraduate with a known history of sickle cell anaemia, presents with a 10-day history of cough, productive of brownish sputum. He has a respiratory rate of 32 cpm and an axillary temperature of 38°C. After clinical assessment an X-ray of the chest, shown here, is obtained.

YOUR TASK:
- To answer the under listed questions using the information from the history and the Chest X-ray provided (Fig 8.3).
- Write your answer on the sheet provided.
- Please drop your answer sheet in the box provided or do as otherwise directed.

TIME ALLOWED: 5 minutes

OSCE Skills for Trainees in Medicine

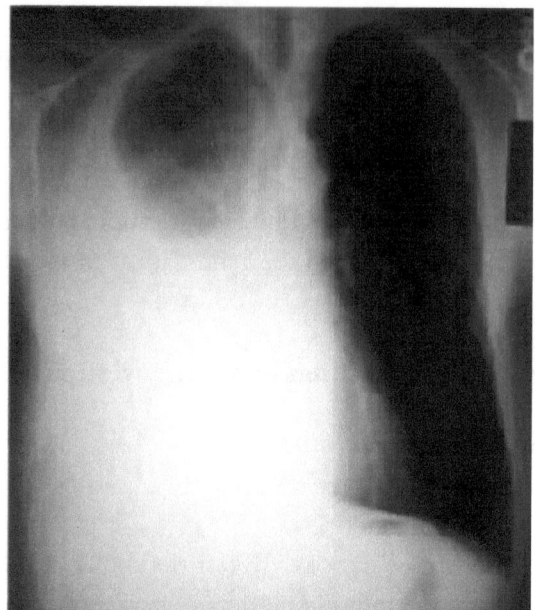

Figure 8.3. Chest X-ray of Yobu at Presentation

Questions on Station X

Answer the following questions based on the history and CXR of the patient.

QUESTION 1. List three important abnormalities on the CXR (3 marks each)

    a. _____
    b. _____
    c. _____

QUESTION 2. What is the radiological diagnosis? (3 marks).

_____

QUESTION 3. What is the most likely underlying condition? (3 marks)

_____

QUESTION 4. List 3 further useful tests in the management of this patient. (3 marks each)

    a. _____
    b. _____
    c. _____

QUESTION 5. List three treatment measures indicated in this patient now (3 marks each)

a. ___ __ ___ _____ __ ___ _____ __ ___ ___
b. ___ __ ___ _____ __ ___ _____ __ ___ ___
c. ___ __ ___ _____ __ ___ _____ __ ___ ___

MODEL ANSWERS FOR GRADING STATION X

QUESTION 1. List 3 important abnormalities on the CXR (Maximum 9 marks)

• Meniscus sign R lung	3 marks
• Homogenous opacity R lung	3 marks
• Mediastinal shift to the left	3 marks
• Tracheal deviation to the left	3 marks
• Right pleural effusion	3 marks
• Cardiomegaly	0 mark
• Consolidation/Pneumonia etc.	0 mark
• Other less important findings	1 mark

QUESTION 2. What is the radiological diagnosis? (Maximum score: 3 marks)

• Right pleural effusion	3 marks
• Pleural effusion	2 marks
• Other	0 mark

QUESTION 3. What is the most likely underlying condition? (Maximum 3 marks)

• Poorly treated lobar pneumonia	3 marks
• Lobar pneumonia	2 marks
• Pneumonia	1 mark
• Heart failure	1 mark
• Sickle cell anaemia	1 mark

QUESTION 4. List 3 further useful tests in this condition (Maximum 9 marks)

- Sputum microscopy and culture — 3 marks
- Pleural aspirate for analysis and culture — 3 marks
- Full blood count and ESR — 3 marks
- Blood gas analysis — 3 marks
- Blood culture — 3 marks
- Pleural biopsy — 1 mark
- Chest CT scan — 1 mark
- Liver function tests — 2 marks
- Sputum for Zn Stain — 1 mark
- Other less important tests — 1 mark

QUESTION 5. List 3 specific treatment measures or agents needed now in this patient. (Maximum Score, 9 marks)

- Intra-nasal oxygen — 3 marks
- Oxygen — 2 marks
- Antibiotics — 1 mark
- Parental antibiotics — 2 marks
- Intravenous appropriate antimicrobial — 3 marks
- Intravenous fluid — 3 marks
- Hospitalisation — 3 marks
- Other less important measures — 1 mark

Total maximum marks: 33 marks Candidate's score: _____

COMMENTS: Note that the station designer (the person who set the question) provides more than the required number of answers but that the options may carry different marks. When answering written questions, therefore, always write your most likely answer first.

8.6.2. Station XIV: Written Post-Encounter Station

Note that in this type of written or *question station*, the task is based on what transpired at the preceding station.

STATIC STATION

General Information
STATION NUMBER: **XIV**
STATION TITLE: Post-encounter station
STATION CONSTRUCT OR PURPOSE: To test the ability of the candidate to identify and interpret physical findings on examination of a patient.

Candidate Briefing and Instructions

SCENARIO: At the (*sic supposedly*) last station, you examined Mr Trego Truman, a 34-year-old man who presented with a fever of three weeks' duration. You were asked to focus the examination on the cardiovascular system.

YOUR TASK: Answer the following questions based on your findings on the history and examination of Mr. Truman. You may refer to the notes you made at the last station.

TIME ALLOWED: 5 minutes

QUESTION 1: *Which of the following were present in the patient? (Answer T/F)*
 a. A pulse deficit
 b. Grade three finger clubbing
 c. Splinter haemorrhages
 d. A grade 4 pansystolic murmur at the apex
 e. A diastolic murmur at the left second intercostal space

QUESTION 2. *Given the history and physical findings, list five investigations that should be performed now in this patient.*
 a. --
 b. --
 c. --
 d. --
 e. --

NB: This question can be made an MCQ type by listing the options for you to identify the correct or incorrect answers.

QUESTION 3. *List four treatment measures that should be taken now in the management of this patient while awaiting results of investigations.*
 a. --

b. --
c. --
d. --

ANSWER TO QUESTION 3

Answer to Question 3 will depend on the case in question. If we assume that the patient has infective endocarditis, what will be the likely answer to this question?

8.6.3. Station XX: Written Station- ECG Quiz

General Information
STATION NUMBER: **XX**
STATION TITLE: Written Station/Data Interpretation
STATION CONSTRUCT OR PURPOSE: To test the ability of the candidate to systematically read and evaluate ECG findings.

Candidate Briefing and Instructions
SCENARIO: Fig 8.4 is the 6 limb-lead ECG of Chief Thomas Cole, a 60-year-old man who complains of breathlessness and chest pain, both of sudden onset.

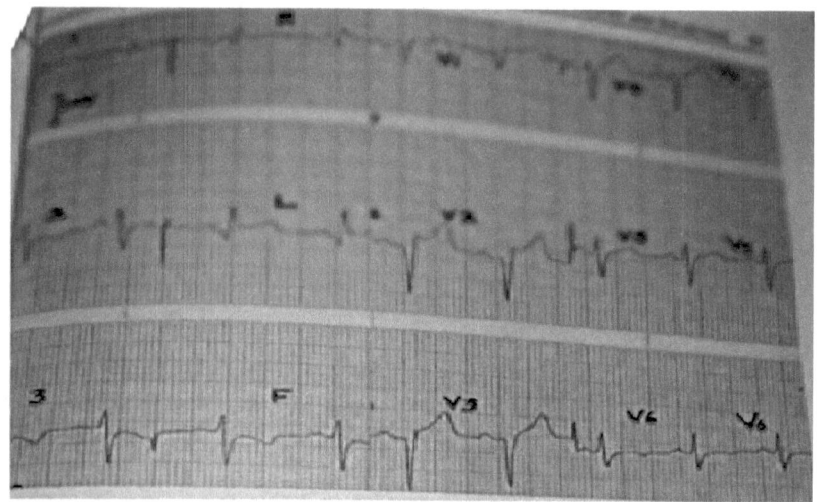

Figure 8.4. ECG Tracing of Thomas Cole

YOUR TASK: *To read the ECG tracing systematically and interpret your findings by answering the questions provided*
TIME ALLOWED: 5 minutes

Station XX Questions
QUESTION 1: *What 5 abnormalities are present on this ECG tracing?*
QUESTION 2: *Given the patient's complaint, what is the most likely cause of these ECG changes?*
QUESTION 3: *List five further tests that are indicated in this patient.*

Station XX: Model Answers
ANSWER TO QUESTIONS 1: *Note the patient details and date of recording.* Systematically provide the following and identify any abnormalities on them:

- Rate
- Axis
- Rhythm
- P wave
- R wave
- PR Interval
- QRS width
- QRS height
- Pathological Q waves
- ST segment
- T waves
- Other

Answers to Questions 2 and 3 will depend on the actual case. The ECG shows classic features of acute myocardial infarction.

8.6.4. Station XXI: Post-encounter (as Short Answer Questions)

General Information
STATION NUMBER: XXI
STATION TITLE: Written Station; Post-encounter Probe (PEP)
STATION CONSTRUCT OR PURPOSE: To test the ability of the candidate to assess a diabetic foot, assess and manage the patient's problem appropriately.

Candidate Briefing and Instructions
PROBLEM/SETTING: At the (*sic presumed*) last station, you examined the feet of Mr John Loga who had had diabetes mellitus for 15 years. You were also asked to record your findings.

YOUR TASK: Answer the following questions based on your findings of the examination of the feet of Mr Loga.
TIME ALLOWED 5 minutes

Questions on Station XXI

QUESTION 1. List three neurological findings present on examination of Mr Loga's feet.
   a. --
   b. --
   c. --

QUESTION 2. Based on your findings describe the class or stage of diabetic foot syndrome to which the feet of Mr Loga belong using the Wagner wound classification system. ------------------------------------

QUESTION 3. Mr Loga is to have surgery of the foot. List three important investigations that would guide the management of his foot problem.
   a. --
   b. --
   c. --

The answer to these question would depend on your findings. You may note however that at the preceding station it is presumed that you methodologically, faithfully and systematically conducted the examination and recorded your findings.

8.6.5. Station XXII. Post-encounter Questions as Multi[le Choice Questions

General Information
STATION NUMBER: XXII
STATION TITLE: Written Station; Post-encounter Probe (PEP)
STATION CONSTRUCT OR PURPOSE: To test the ability of the candidate to assess cardiac status and manage the patient's problem appropriately.

STATIC STATION

Station XXII: Candidate Instructions

PROBLEM/SETTING: At the last station you examined the heart of Ms Alice Wong.

YOUR TASK: Answer the following questions based on your findings of the examination of Ms Wong at the last station.

Questions on Station XXII (Select the single best answer)

QUESTION 1: Which of the following physical signs **were** present in the patient?

i. A soft first heart sound
ii. An ejection systolic murmur at the base of the heart
iii. A rumbling diastolic murmur
iv. An opening snap
v. A pansystolic murmur at the apex radiating to the axilla

Indicate which ONE of the following combinations is correct about the findings in the patient

a. i and ii
b. ii and iii
c. iii and iv
d. iv and v
e. ii and v

QUESTION 2. Which one of the following would best explain the physical findings in the patient?

a. Mitral stenosis
b. Mitral incompetence
c. Aortic stenosis
d. Aortic regurgitation
e. Mitral prolapse

QUESTION 3. Based on your findings, which of the following tests **are** indicated in this patient now? Select the single best answer from the test combinations options a-e.

i. Resting 12 lead ECG tracing
ii. Stress ECG test
iii. Echocardiography

iv. Plain Chest X-ray
v. Estimation of plasma levels of troponin C

Select the best combination of tests needed:
a. i, iii, and iv
b. ii, iii, and iv
c. iii, iv, and v
d. i, iv, and v
e. ii, iv, and v

8.7. CHAPTER EIGHT SUMMARY

- There are two main types of active stations in an OSPE/OSCE exercise: *interactive stations* manned by examiners and *non-interactive or written station*s which have no examiner physically present there.
- Several competencies such as patient management, data and image interpretation, written communication, and clinical reasoning can be assessed at the *written station*.
- Question formats at the written station include short answer questions, completion questions, labelling, and MCQs.
- When asked to provide a number of options, start with the most important one. If asked for two causes, give two and no more.
- Ensure you understand what is required of you at the station; read the instructions carefully before you answer the question.

8.8. CHAPTER EIGHT RECAP EXERCISES

1. How is the written station different from the other types of stations in an OSCE/OSPE circuit?
2. List five competencies assessable using pen and paper in the OSCE/OSPE.
3. Concerning written stations, indicate whether *True or False*
   a. It is better to mention more than the required number of responses to a given question.
   b. If asked to list causes of a disorder, start from the most likely to the least likely.
4. Regarding usage of written stations

a. Name two advantages in using written stations for assessment.
b. Name two limitations in using written stations for assessment.
5. Create one practice question for a written station. Provide model answers.

8.9. Bibliography and Resources. See page 249

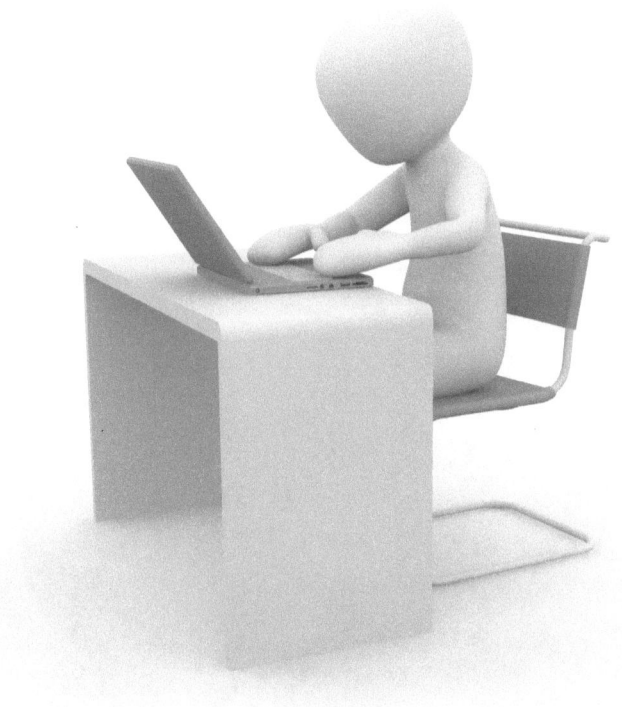

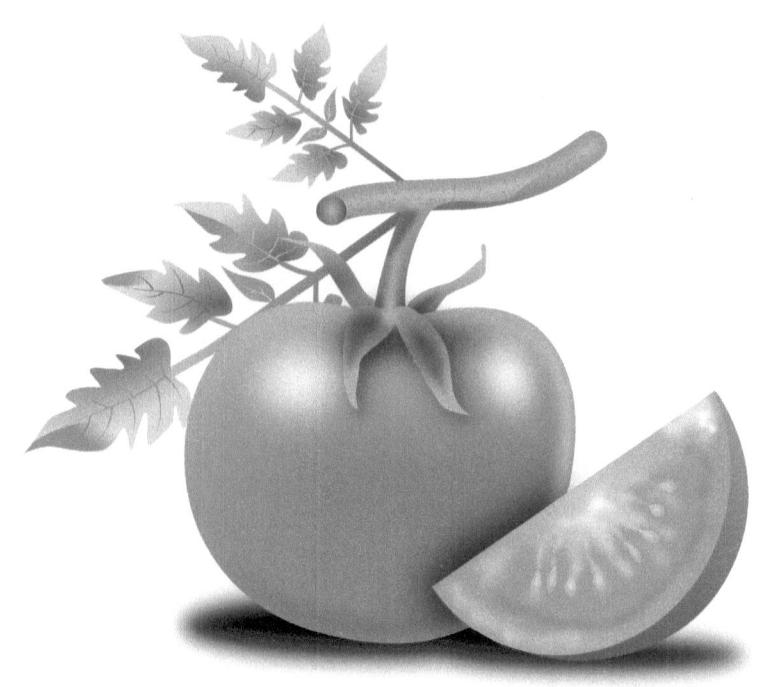

9

Structured Viva Voce Station

9.1. Introduction

9.2. Purpose of *Viva Voce*

9.3. Merits and Drawbacks of Traditional Orals

9.4. Structured *Viva Voce Examination*

9.5. Competencies Assessable at a Structured *Viva*

9.6. The Process of a Structured *Viva Voce*

9.7. Elements at a Structured *Viva* Station

9.8. Format of Questions at a Structured *Viva* Station

9.9. An Example of a Structured *Viva Voce* Station

9.10. Advice on Handling Structured Orals

9.11 Chapter Nine Summary

9.12. Chapter Nine Recap Exercises

9.13. Bibliography and Resources

9.14. Appendices

9.1. INTRODUCTION

Traditional *viva voce* also often referred to as *oral examination* used to be an integral part of the standard approach in assessing undergraduate and postgraduate trainees in many medical fields. In recent years oral examinations have come under severe criticisms such that they are being abandoned by many examining bodies and schools but some traditionalists still use them. *Viva voce* as an assessment tool, in spite of its many limitations, has some advantages over other tools. It appears that *Viva voce* will continue to be in use for some time. You should, therefore, be prepared to face one when the need arises.

The good news for the candidate is that efforts are being made to improve the use of oral examinations in the spirit of OSCE; the structured format that is more examinee-friendly and more objective has been introduced. Before discussing structured oral examination *per se* let's see why some examiners continue to insist on retaining the oral examination as a tool in assessment of medical trainees.

9.2. PURPOSE OF *VIVA VOCE*

A traditional oral examination consists of a dialogue between the candidate and one or more examiners who ask questions, usually of their own choosing. The questions, which often vary between candidates, are meant to probe whether the students can express their knowledge of facts or groups of facts they ought to remember. Scoring the oral examination by using multiple examiners tends to settle on averaging examiners' scores.

Proponents of oral examinations often quote what the great philosopher, Plato, had to say about oral and written methods of assessment:

> *Writing would destroy the need for memory; students would receive information but without proper instruction and would therefore appear to be knowledgeable while in fact being quite ignorant. On the other hand, the spoken word "is written on the soul of the hearer with understanding", and the written word is only a pale shadow of "the living and animate speech of a man with knowledge"* (Phaedrus).

9.3. MERITS AND DRAWBACKS OF TRADITIONAL ORALS

There are several reasons arguably in favour of using oral assessment in medical education (See Table 9.1) The downside of orals includes the issues listed in Table 9.1.

Table 9.1. Merits and Drawbacks of Traditional Orals

Drawbacks	Merits
• Can be threatening and stressful to the candidate.	• Allows examiner to give hints to elicit the desired responses and memory blocks can be cleared.
• Majority of questions are of the recall type.	
• Orals may bias against some candidates	• Allow probing of the students' knowledge in depth.
• Outcome may depend on the emotional state of the candidate such as anxiety, tension, apprehension etc.	• At one session, orals can assess a student's progression from "Reporter" through "Interpreter" to "Manager/ Educator" (RIME).
• Questions frequently vary from student to student and from one examiner to another; thus some students may get easy questions while others get difficult ones.	• May give flexibility to the examiner to move from strong to weak areas and vice versa at one session.
• Tend to assess certain attributes which are not intended to be assessed; e.g. examinee's style of speaking.	• Meaning of questions can be more easily clarified in orals.
• Time consuming and expensive	• Orals can be comprehensive and offer feedback.
• Traditional oral questions lack standardization.	• Orals appear to reflect the world of practice.
• Undue influence of irrelevant factors, such as "halo" effect,	• Plato argued strongly in its favour
• Very time-consuming and an expensive	

There appears to be some strong argument for the continued use of oral examination in assessment of students in the health professions. However, there are more compelling reasons why oral examination should not be used in the traditional format due to its many drawbacks. The solution appears to be the adoption of the structured form of oral examinations.

9.4. STRUCTURED *VIVA VOCE* EXAMINATION

One of the recent major modifications of the traditional *viva voce* has been the attempt to streamline the questions asked and objectify the grading of answers through the use of a *structured approach* to the examination. This modified oral examination can be used in addition to or as part of a multi-station OSCE. The use of structured *viva voce* is one of the best ways to correct the poor inter-examiner reliability and poor objectivity of traditional oral examinations.

Format of a Structured Oral Examination

A structured oral examination (SOE) typically consists of sequential presentation of pre-determined scenarios of a clinical case or problem. Such a scenario has a set of four to six questions attached to it, each with a specific marking scheme. The student is presented with the clinical scenario or problem and is then asked a number of questions going systematically. The SOE station is usually manned and assessed by two independent examiners.

The Merits and Drawbacks of Structured *Viva Voce*

Some of the advantages of using a structured, standardised oral examination (SOE) as well as some of the limitations are:

MERITS OF USING A STRUCTURED ORAL EXAMINATION
- Structured oral examination (SOE) can be used to assess aspects of trainees that other examination formats may fail to assess.
- SOE can assess the candidate's cognitive abilities related to clinical practice, such as problem solving and decision making.
- SOE approach helps to ensure that all the examinees receive a similar form of assessment, in terms of content, outcomes, item difficulty and examiner leniency.
- SOE can be used to assess the candidate's cognitive abilities related to clinical practice, such as problem solving and decision making.

DRAWBACKS OF STRUCTURED ORAL EXAMINATION
- Structured oral examinations are difficult to design.
- If not properly designed the test can become an exercise in factual recall.

STRUCTURED ORALS

- The SOE approach is manpower intensive.
- The emotional state of the candidate may influence the outcome of SOE
- Some of the demerits of traditional viva may still operate.

An important characteristic of SOE is that it can deploy many clinical scenarios on which to base assessment/ judgement. Failing the station does not depend on being unlucky with the questions or the idiosyncrasy of a particular examiner. However, the SOE has its own drawbacks too. The SOE is not a perfect system but its merits appear to far outweigh its limitations and it is likely to receive more acceptance and patronage in the future. More and more examiners are likely to be using it; therefore be familiar with how the system works and the type of competencies it is most suited for.

9.5. SKILLS ASSESSABLE AT A STRUCTURED *VIVA*

The SOE can be used to assess a large number of competencies such as:
- Personal qualities; e.g. attitudes, personality, integrity, demeanour
- Communication skills
- Professionalism
- Surgical experience
- Ability to integrate competencies
- Organisation and logical, step-wise sequencing of the thought process;
- Ability to focus on the answer quickly
- Ability to justify an answer with evidence from the literature
- Clinical reasoning, decision making skills, and prioritisation
- Adaptability to stress and ability to handle stress
- Ability to deal with 'grey areas' in practice and complex issues not be easily assessed by other methods.

An SOE may be case-based or problem-based. In a case-based SOE, a patient scenario is introduced and questions on presentation, diagnosis, and management are asked sequentially. In a problem-based session, a theme is presented followed by management questions; for example: heart failure; child in sickle cell pain crisis, hypokalaemia, shock etc.

9.6. THE PROCESS OF A STRUCTURED *VIVA*

The SOE process, in summary, runs according to a sequence like as follows:

- Examiner: An introductory statement (about a patient) is presented. Examiner asks a question on available information.
- *The candidate answers and examiners score.*
- Examiner gives candidate further information and Examiner asks further questions based on the new information e.g. what are your differential diagnoses?
- *The candidate answers.*
- Examiner continues, providing more data /results of tests related to the case and Examiner asks candidate more focused questions such as: What is your final diagnosis?
- *Candidate answers*
- Examiner poses more probing questions
- *Candidate answers*
- More probing questions are asked.
- *Candidate continues to answer*

Types of Questions at a Structured Viva

The questions asked at an SOE station may be broadly grouped into four technical types: introductory questions focus questions, competency questions, and default or escape questions. The introductory question is usually simple and is such that most candidates will get it right. The focus question is directed at what is to be discussed. The competency question, the main object of the station, is more difficult and sets off more probing questions and some discussion. Each of these categories of questions may contain subsections.

Default and *escape questions* which are very simple but non-scoring are asked when candidates are unable to answer a scoring question and there is need to move to the next questions without making the candidate feel demoralised. However, note that the examiner does not have to tell you what type of question you are being asked.

9.7. ELEMENTS AT A *VIVA VOCE* STATION

Examiners at a Structured Viva Station

An SOE station is similar to a communications or history station with one major difference: the station is directly driven by the examiner. Neither patients nor assistants are usually present at an SOE station, just you and the examiners (see Figure 9.1), one of whom may be designated the lead examiner for a particular candidate. Interaction between the candidate and the examiners is rather much more extensive than at any other OSCE station. The examiner may talk for about 20% or less of the time while the candidate should be talking for about 80% of the time.

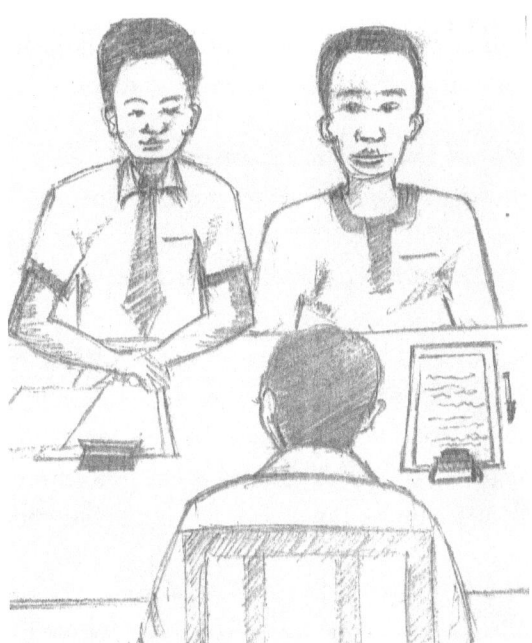

Figure 9.1. A Viva Voce Setting. *Almost any questions may be asked at a viva station. You are facing one or more examiners and popular **frequently asked questions** are hurled at you. Effective communication associated with substance is required of you here. Always think before answering.*

Information Items at the SOE Station

At the Structured Oral Examination (SOE) station there are general information and instructions about what is to be done at the station. Among such information items at an SOE station are the following:

- General station elements (station title, station number, and station purpose).
- Patient scenario presented in phases by the examiner
- Candidate instructions
- Examiner instructions
- Questions with model answers of varying degrees of accuracy
- Scoring sheet and instructions
- Task-specific requirements such as a viewing box, a printout, an instrument, lab data etc. may be provided
- Feedback forms

Of all these station elements, the first three items should be the ones of immediate interest to the candidate at the examination but you should also have some idea of what the other items are about.

General Structured Viva Station Elements

The *Station Title or Type* gives the broad competency domain to be examined at the station. Here it may be stated as Structured Viva or Structured Oral Examination. The *Station Number* is shown on each station document. *Station Construct* describes the purpose of the station: e.g. the purpose of this station is to assess the ability of the candidate to read and interpret a CT scan; to interpret data and manage a case, etc. The construct may be incorporated into the candidate's instruction. The *Stem or Scenario* refers to the background to the problem to be tackled by the candidate. It is usually cast in a few lines and is easily understandable.

Information and Instructions for the Candidate

The way an SOE system works is rather different from the other OSCE stations. Both the candidate and the examiners should therefore have had a pre-examination experience such as in a formative SOE. You will need to exhibit your clinical reasoning ability and how to go about progressively solving a clinical problem. The opening candidate information may be structured like as follows:

STATION NUMBER: Station X
STATION TITLE: Structured Oral Examination
STATION CONSTRUCT OR PURPOSE: Chosen competency domain

PATIENT SCENARIO: You are a (specified grade) staff in a (specified) health facility. The patient of specified demographics presents with a history of a (specified) symptom.

YOUR TASK: Your task is to listen to and follow the examiners as they provide graduated information about the patient and to answer the questions they will put to you.

TIME ALLOWED: 5/10/15 minutes as determined by the rules.

Guide on Examining at an SOE station

Generally an SOE station will be manned by two examiners especially at postgraduate examinations. The examiners must have been extensively briefed about the station and the SOE process. The examiner would, for each phase of the scenario, ask the relevant structured question (introductory *questions, focus questions, or competency question*). He reads the initial presentation of the patient (or allows you to read it yourself) and then asks a clear question such as "what will you do next?" or presents results of initial tests and asks "what will you do next?" or "Interpret these results". He should end the session by asking or reading the *competency question*, the thrust of the station as indicated in the construct. If the candidate gets stuck, the examiner will ask a simple *default* or *escape* question to move the process forward.

The examiner scores each phase of the question independently in addition to providing a global rating. Both you and the examiner have to ensure that you go through all the "scoring" questions at the station. Therefore, *avoid time wasting actions*. For any question not attempted, you would be scored zero. The examiner is enjoined to avoid leading questions and should not give unplanned cues to any student except for any prompts previously agreed to by all examiners

Test Materials at a Structured *Viva* Station

At the SOE there may be instruments, lab results, patient scenarios etc. depending on the purpose and subject matter of the station. Such materials are used to drive the interaction between the candidate and the examiners, see Figure 9.2.

OSCE Skills for Trainees in Medicine

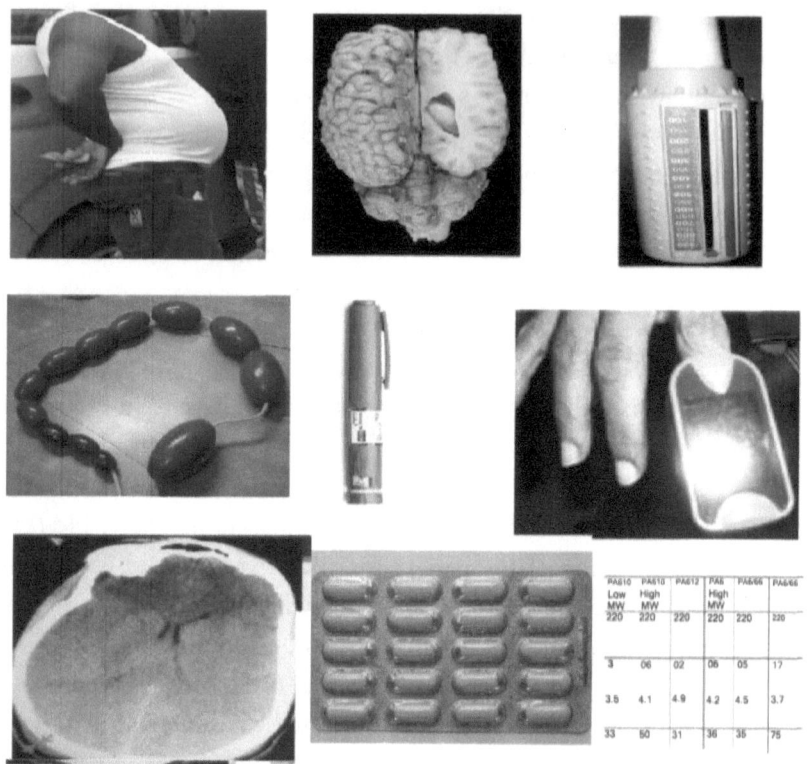

Figure 9.2. Materials and Themes for a Structured Oral Examination. *Almost any materials can be used to kick start a viva. Tasks under written and practical procedure stations can be readily deployed for this purpose. Think of themes for questioning to which the materials here might put.*

9.8. FORMAT OF QUESTIONS AT A STRUCTURED *VIVA* STATION

As mentioned earlier there are four main types of questions you might be asked at the SOE station although you will not be told what type of question you are being asked: *introductory questions, focus questions, competency questions, and default or escape questions.*

Introductory Question

The first or *introductory question* asked at SOE station follows directly from the clinical scenario or problem presented and is usually easy to answer. The examiner will read out the introductory question *verbatim* to the candidate.

Default and Escape Questions

Default and Escape Questions are very simple questions that are asked only if the candidate gets stuck with *a scoring question*. These are soft landing questions! The answer to the *default question* carries no marks. The last default question asked at the station is often referred to as *escape question,* to end the station interaction.

Focus Question

After dealing with the introductory question, more information is provided to the candidate and a *Focus Question* (**FQ**), which narrows the scene down towards the major point of interest to be addressed, is posed. There may be more than one focus question asked for each stem. A second *default question*, a very simple question, may be asked if the candidate gets stuck with the *Focus Question*.

Competency Question

The *competency question* (CQ) is an advanced question to test the candidate's grasp of the specific issue under discussion. This question should reveal whether the candidate is "safe" to deal with the clinical problem. The examiner engages the candidate in a limited discussion around the CQ. An escape question (**EQ**) is the last easy parting question that is posed only if the candidate gets stuck with the *competency question*. The EQ like the *default question* carries no marks but should leave the candidate psychologically better off as he moves to the next station.

Note that default and escape questions are non-scoring and are only asked if a candidate runs into difficulty with the real questions. However you will not be told which are scoring or default questions but you might be able to guess. Good candidates won't get asked this type of soft landing questions.

9.9. AN EXAMPLE OF A STRUCTURED *VIVA VOCE* STATION

Remember that the essential parts of the station are the General Information about the station, the Scenarios, and the Questions. Model answers are provided for the use of the examiners.

9.9.1. STATION XXIII

General Information about the Station
    STATION NUMBER: XXIII
    STATION TITLE: Structured *Viva Voce*
    TIME ALLOWED: 10 minutes
    STATION CONSTRUCT: The purpose of the station is to test the candidate's ability to perform, and interpret the results of an OGTT in pregnancy.

Information and Instructions to Candidate
Please carefully read the following information about the station and the Instructions to the Candidate. You may make notes.
    STATION TITLE: Structured *Viva Voce*
    TIME ALLOWED: 10 minutes
    STATION CONSTRUCT: The purpose of this station is to test your ability to evaluate a woman with poor obstetric history.
    SCENARIO AND PROCESS: Tena Kowo, a 26-year-old woman with a history of recurrent abortions presents to the antennal clinic where you are a registrar in a firm. The examiner will provide you with clinical and laboratory data about the woman and ask you how you will manage each scenario. The examiner will provide the information in stages or chunks and then ask you some questions based on the information available. Following that they will provide you with more information and ask you further questions. The process continues this way until you get to the last question or time expires.
    YOUR TASK: Your task is to listen to and follow the examiners as they provide graduated information about the patient and to answer the questions they will put to you.

Scenarios and Questions

Scenario Phase I
    INFORMATION. A woman complains of frequent miscarriages. She is para 0+ 3, all miscarriages occurred in the third trimester. She is now 16 weeks pregnant.

STRUCTURED ORALS

QUESTION 1. *What initial three endocrine tests are indicated in this patient?*

DEFAULT QUESTION. *What two common endocrine conditions adversely affect pregnancy outcome?* (Asked only if candidate is unable to answer Q1.)

Scenario Phase II

INFORMATION. On initial investigation the following results were obtained; (Examiner hands you a paper with the results): *Glycosuria, 2+; Proteinuria, nil; Ketonuria, absent Fasting plasma glucose (FPG), 99 mg/dl (5.5 mmol/l).*

QUESTION 2. *How do you interpret these results?*

DEFAULT QUESTION. *What can cause glycosuria in pregnancy?* (Asked only if candidate is unable to answer Question 2.

Scenario Phase III

INFORMATION (From Examiner). With these results we suspect what the diagnosis should be. There is a need to confirm our diagnosis.

QUESTION 3. *In the further management of this patient, which one confirmatory test will you like to perform and why?*

DEFAULT QUESTION. *In pregnant patients with diabetes mellitus, is HbA1C a good reflection of glycaemia?* (Asked only if candidate is unable to answer Q3.)

Scenario Phase IV

INFORMATION. When basal blood glucose levels are equivocal, we have to perform an OGTT to make a diagnosis of diabetes mellitus (DM). Therefore, it was decided that the patient should have an OGTT.

QUESTION 4. *Describe how an OGTT is performed using the WHO guidelines in a pregnant woman.*

DEFAULT QUESTION. *Will 24-hour quantification of glycosuria be helpful in the work-up of this patient?* (Asked only if candidate is unable to answer Q4.)

OSCE Skills for Trainees in Medicine

Table 9. 2. Marksheet for Structured Viva Voce Station XXIII

Item	
	Q1. List three initial endocrine tests indicated in this patient? (Maximum subtotal score 7 marks)
1 to 3	a. Urinalysis for glucose, ketones, and proteinuria 0-1-2-3
	b. Casual blood glucose: 2 marks
	c. Fasting plasma glucose (FPG): 2 marks
	d. 2 h-post-prandial plasma glucose level: 2 marks
	e. HbA1C: 1 mark
	f. other answer: 0 mark
	Q2. How do you interpret the results? (Maximum subtotal score, 10 marks)
4	a. FPG within normal limits but too high in pregnant state: 0- 1 - 2
	b. Glycosuria suggests DM but in pregnancy, renal glucosuria is common (lowering of renal threshold for glucose and should not be used to make diagnosis of gestational DM (GDM) 0 - 1 – 2
	c. Asks what reagent was used for the test (as copper sulphate-based reagents produce false positive results). 0 - 1 – 2
	d. Explains why the glucose tolerance status cannot be determined from these results: 0 - 1 – 2
	e. Suggests patient possibly has GDM 0 - 1 – 2
	Q 3. Which ONE confirmatory test will you like to do and why? 0 - 1 - 2 - 3- 4- 5 (Maximum score:5 marks)
5	a. OGTT with 75 g glucose for 2 h (WHO) *or*
	b. 100 g for 3 hours (O'Sullivan) 0 - 1 - 2 - 3- 4- 5
	c. 50 g glucose and 1 h PGL 1 – 2 marks
	d. Repeat FPG 1 mark
	e. HbA1C 1 mark
	f. Any other 0
	Q 4. How is OGTT performed using the WHO guidelines in a pregnant woman. (Maximum subtotal score 21 marks)
6	a. Prepare patient; including diet, fasting overnight, 8-12 h: 0 - 1 - 2 – 3
	b. Rest the patient on arrival: 0 - 1 – 2
	c. Prepare GOD bottles: labels etc.: 0 - 1 – 2
	d. Withdraw venous blood at 0 min for FPG: 0 - 1 – 2
	e. Give 75 g anhydrous glucose: 0 - 1 - 2 3
	f. In 250-300 ml water: 0 - 1 - 2- 3

Table 9. 2. Marksheet for Structured Viva Voce Station XXIII

	g. Solution ingested in about 3 min **0 – 2 – 3**
	h. Withdraw venous blood again at 120 min. 0 - 1 - 2 – 3
	Question 5: What is your interpretation of the OGTT results? (Maximum subtotal score: 10 marks)
7	a. FPG is high normal 0 – 1 – 2
	b. 2-h PGL is higher than normal but lower than DM cut-off for non pregnant state. 0 - 1 – 2
	c. The OGTT plasma glucose pattern is impaired glucose tolerance (IGT) or prediabetes in non-pregnant state 0 - 1 – 2
	d. In pregnancy, IGT is regarded as GDM 0 - 1 – 2
	e. The patient should be treated as case of GDM 0 - 1 – 2
	Question 6. So this pregnant woman with this level of plasma glucose level should be treated as if she has GDM. What is the evidence for this line of management? (Maximum subtotal score 5 marks)
8	ANSWER: Discusses how any degree of elevation in plasma glucose level is deleterious to the foetus. 0 - 1 - 2 - 3 -4-5
9	Total Score
10	Global Rating Excellent; Good; Borderline; Fail; Very Poor
	Comments
	Name Signature Date

Scenario Phase V

INFORMATION. The plasma glucose levels during the OGTT were as follows (examiner hands over the test results to you):

Fasting plasma glucose (FPG): 108 mg/dl (6 mmol/l) –
2-h post-glucose load (PGL): 180 mg/dl (10 mmol/l)

QUESTION 5. *What is your interpretation of the results of this OGTT?*

ESCAPE QUESTION. *Which is more reliable to diagnose diabetes mellitus: urine sugar or OGTTNINE? (Asked only if the candidate is unable to answer Q5.)*

Scenario Phase VI: SHORT DISCUSSION OR PROBING
INFORMATION FROM EXAMINER. In pregnancy, a plasma glucose level not in the diabetes range but higher than normal as in this woman should be treated as if the pregnant woman had diabetes mellitus.
QUESTION 6. *What is the evidence for this line of management?*
ESCAPE QUESTION. *What are the risks to the foetus in a pregnant woman with diabetes in pregnancy?* (Asked only if candidate is unable to answer Q6)

Model Answers to Questions

Note that these questions are provided with answers of varying degrees of correctness. The most correct answer gets the maximum marks available. Of course this information will not be available to you at the station. We are providing it to help you when you meet similar scenarios in the future.

Instructions to the Examiner

Please score the candidate appropriately as in Table 9.2, giving the maximum mark if the answer is adequate, midway mark if answer is just fair and lower or no mark if answer is wrong or not provided.

9.10. ADVICE ON TACKLING STRUCTURED ORALS

Many candidates think of the SOE station as being very difficult. This is not necessarily true. Characteristic of the OSCE approach to assessment, the questions tend to be fair. The examiners follow the written script and should not deviate from it. The following hints and tips might help you to improve your performance at the SOE station, if you have to face one.

1. As at every OSCE station, read the instruction and scenario information at the SOE station very carefully.
2. If asked a question, ensure you understand the questions before answering.
3. Demonstrate a systematic approach to answering the questions; suggest appropriate management or further investigations when asked.
4. Unlike a traditional *viva voce*, SOE is a fair situation; the examiners are not allowed to ask any question they like as they have a rigid

list of questions/topics through which they have to guide you; just follow their instructions.

5. Put on your *listening cap*; listen carefully before answering. If a question put orally is not clear to you, politely ask for a repeat or clarification.
6. Avoid arguing with the examiner or wasting time in any way as the more material covered by you the more marks you are likely to garner. If you do not know the answer to a question, be honest and tell the examiner so that you can move on. The examiners go on to a different topic if you appear to be stalling or looking blank.
7. We all fear the hawkish examiner but here the harm they can inflict on you is limited as their hands are tied by the predetermined scenarios, questions, and answers. Nothing can be fairer if you have played your own part.
8. Practise often before the examination; request your seniors and peers (and even peers) to drill you frequently.
9. Appear confident. Try to avoid wild gesticulations and nervous habits or murmuring to yourself. Avoid mentioning subjects about which your knowledge is shallow as you may get stuck when probed deeper. Struggling with answers tends to whittle down your confidence and esteem.
10. When asked a question, do not rush to answer even if you think you know. Take a few seconds to think about the question - i.e. what the examiner requires. Do not give your answers in the form of questions to the examiner. Many examiners get put off by answers put as questions such as "Can it be pneumonia?"
11. If asked to identify abnormalities, describe the most 'obvious' abnormality first before discussing the other ones.
12. Know what your limitations are. Say when a problem should be passed on to a senior but you should be able to make your own plan if faced with a problem. However, do not just pass all problems to others!
13. Try get to be asked all the scoring questions at the station. Do not waste time unnecessarily as you have to go over all the aspects of the question for you to score maximally. For questions you do not

get to before the bell goes, those marks are all lost as you will be awarded no marks.
14. Do not damage or write on the question sheet passed onto you.
15. Always be polite to the examiner.
16. Try and sound as professional and confident as possible, and speak clearly. Introduce yourself as you enter, and say - 'Thank you, Sir or Ma'... as you leave.
17. Questions proceed down a designated pathway involving various aspects of a patient's care. The examiners expect you to follow this pathway for you to score maximally. Follow the cues, if any, from the examiner.
18. You are not supposed to be asked questions that are not specified by the scenario, but some examiners may still do so. If you are asked questions that appear not to refer to the scenario, keep calm and answer them as best as you can. They may be *default questions* which are usually simple.
19. Remember, if a particular question goes awry, do not panic, there are many more chances. Move on quickly to the next question and do not dwell on past mistakes.
20. Again, Remember to thank the examiners as you take leave of them!

9.11. CHAPTER NINE SUMMARY

- Traditional oral examinations have poor reliability and are being replaced with structured oral examinations (SOE) which can be made part of an OSCE/OSPE exercise.
- The SOE process consists of providing information about a problem or patient in phases to the candidate. There is a predetermined path the discussion is to go and the candidate is expected to find themselves along this pathway.
- For each set of information provided to the candidate relevant questions are asked. If the candidate cannot answer the question, a simple alternative one which is non-scoring is asked.
- It is important that you move fast enough to attempt all questions and garner the maximum marks you can from the station.

9.12. CHAPTER NINE RECAP EXERCISES
1. What did Plato say about *viva voce*?
2. List three merits and one limitation of the use of a Structured Oral Examination (SOE).
3. List five competencies that SOE can be used to assess?
4. List four classes of questions that may be used at an SOE station.
5. Suggest three scenarios or problems in your specialty that might be appropriate for an SOE station.

9.13. BIBLIOGRAPHY AND RESOURCES, see page 249

9.14. APPENDICES

Appendix 9.1 Potential Tasks For Structured *Viva*

- Applied Biochemistry
- Applied clinical pharmacology
- Applied physiology
- Clinical measurement
- Communication skills, attitudes and behaviour
- Day surgery
- Diagnostic imaging
- Anaesthesia and sedation
- Evidence based medicine
- Generic knowledge and skills
- Healthcare Management
- Infection control
- Intensive and high dependency care
- Intra-operative care (including sedation)
- Management of respiratory and cardiac arrest
- Trauma and accidents
- Medical Ethics and Law
- Obstetric anaesthesia
- Ophthalmic anaesthesia
- Orthopaedic anaesthesia
- Pain management: acute and chronic
- Performance of procedures
- Postoperative and recovery care
- Premedication
- Preoperative assessment
- Regional anaesthesia
- Research /Publications
- Statistical basis of clinical trial management
- Statistical methods
- Teaching and medical education
- The responsibilities of a professional

Appendix 9.2. Example of a Problem- Based SOE Station

General Information about Station

STATION TITLE: Structured Viva Voce

STATION CONSTRUCT: To test the ability of the candidate to manage a case of hyponatraemia

SCENARIO. Mr James Peters is a 70-year-old man being managed for behavioural problems that started about three weeks before presentation. Blood work-up shows electrolyte abnormalities which need to be managed appropriately.

Briefing and Instructions to the Candidate

STRUCTURED ORALS

PURPOSE. The purpose of this station is to test your knowledge of, and ability to effectively manage, a common electrolyte disorder.

STATION FORMAT. The station will be run in a structured viva format. The examiner will take you through a series of the patient's scenarios and ask you question/s on each of the scenarios.

SCENARIO. Mr James Peters is a 70-year-old man being managed for behavioural problems that started about three weeks before presentation. Blood work-up shows electrolyte abnormalities which need to managed appropriately.

YOUR TASK. You are the Senior Registrar under whom Mr Peters is admitted. You are to follow the lead examiner's instructions.

TIME ALLOWED: 10 minutes

Information for the Station Examiner

STATION CONSTRUCT. The purpose of this encounter is to assess the ability of the candidate as a Senior Registrar to manage a case of hyponatraemia.

Please read the instructions to the candidates.

STATION FORMAT.

- The station should be run in a structured *viva* manner.
- The lead examiner reads out the scenario and/or shows same to the candidate.
- The candidate responds, examiners score using the marksheet.
- The co-examiner keeps track of the time in addition to scoring

DEFAULT OR ESCAPE QUESTION. If the candidate appears to get stuck or says he does not know, the examiner reads out the simple (non-scoring) *default question* and then moves on to the next scenario/question.

SCORING CANDIDATE'S PERFORMANCE AT VIVA VOCE

a. Use the marksheet to score the accuracy of the answers provided by the candidate.
b. Where answers to questions are weighted, the most accurate answer should attract the maximum marks and less accurate ones decreasing marks.

OSCE Skills for Trainees in Medicine

c. *Independent scoring by team of examiners.* Co-examiners should not discuss performance of any candidate before scoring. Examiners should award marks independently. At the end of the examination the examiner should add up the scores for each candidate.

d. *Global Rating.* Besides scoring each individual answer, the **station** examiner should provide a global rating of the candidate's performance. This should be done before adding the total analytical scores of the candidate. *The global rating should be scored before or at the departure of the candidate from the station.*

e. The general rules concerning the conduct of this examination apply equally to this station.

Scenarios and Questions (For the Station Examiner)

SCENARIO I

Mr James Peters is a 70-year old man being managed for behavioural problems that started about three weeks before presentation. Blood work-up shows electrolyte abnormalities which need to be managed appropriately.

Following the presentation, the following lab serum reports were obtained:
Urea: 3.5 mmol/l Creatinine: 85µmol/l
Sodium: 115 mmol/l Potassium: 3.5 mmol/l
Chloride: 95 mmol/l Bicarbonate: 20 mmol/l

QUESTION 1. *What is the most striking abnormality in these results? (3 marks)*

DEFAULT QUESTION. *Is the sodium level low*

SCENARIO II

After further assessment, it is decided that some more routine tests be undertaken.

QUESTION 2. *Which three further tests will you recommend at this stage to confirm the presence of hyponatraemia? (9 marks)*

DEFAULT QUESTION: *Is salivary sodium determination needed in this man?*

SCENARIO III

Repeat serum electrolytes and urea are essentially unchanged. Other results are as follows:

Total protein: 75g/l
Total cholesterol 3.4 mmol/l
Fasting plasma glucose: 7.1 mmol/l
CXR and FBC: normal

Albumin: 40 g/l
Urine sodium: 80 mmol/l
Repeat plasma urea: 2.8 mmol/l

QUESTION 3
  a. What two abnormalities are present in the latest results? (Maximum score: 4 marks)
  b. What is the significance of these levels of lipids and proteins in this patient? (Maximum score: 5 marks)

DEFAULT QUESTION: *Is it necessary to do a urine culture in this patient?*

SCENARIO IV
On reviewing the patient after several days in hospital the following features are found:

Confused. No pedal or sacral oedema. Pulse rate 84/min and BP 140/85mmHg.

Repeat further test results include the following:
Urine sodium: 60 mmol/l   FPG: 5 mmol/l
Plasma urea: 3.8 mmol/l   Plasma sodium: 111 mmol/l
                              Plasma potassium: 4.0 mmol/l

QUESTION 4
  a. What is the calculated plasma osmolality of the patient? (Maximum score: 5 marks)
  b. There are three main types of hyponatraemia based on plasma sodium and the fluid status. Name the three types. (Maximum score: marks 3)
  c. To which of these classes does this patient belong? Give two justifications for your choice. (Maximum score: 5 marks)

DEFAULT QUESTION: Do the findings suggest hyperosmolar state?

OSCE Skills for Trainees in Medicine

Scenario V
With hyponatraemia and its type established, confirmatory tests need to be done.

Question 5
a. Taking all the available information together, list three differential diagnoses of the hyponatraemia in this patient?.(Maximum 4 marks)
b. State one confirmatory test of the cause of the hyponatraemia for your most likely diagnosis. (Maximum score: 2 marks)

3. Justify the choice of your test. (3 marks)

Default Question. *Why should urinalysis be done in this patient?*

Scenario VI
While awaiting results of further tests, the patient is reported to be more confused and has a seizure.

Question 6. *Mention and discuss briefly three immediate measures and precautions you will now take in the management of this patient. (Max score 15 marks)*

Escape Question. *Will phenytoin be helpful in arresting the seizures?*

Total Score -

Global Rating Excellent; Good; Borderline; Fail; Very Poor
*Candidate reade r may try provide the answers to the questions here.

10

Practical Assessment of Clinical Examination Skills

10.1. Introduction

10.2. Overview of Practical Assessment of Clinical Examination Skills

10.3. Structure and Procedure of PACES

10.4. Comparison of OSCE and PACES

10.5. PACES Criteria for Assessing Performance

10.6. Attributes of a Good Performance

10.7. Advice for the PACES Candidate

10.8. Chapter 10 Summary

10.9. Chapter 10 Recap Exercises

10.1. INTRODUCTION

Since the introduction of OSCE in the 1970's many modifications have been made to it in an attempt to overcome some of its shortcomings or use for other purposes. These attempts have resulted in several variants of OSCE such as Objective Structured Practical Examination (OSPE), Objective Structured Long Case Examination Records (OSLER), and **P**ractical Assessment of **C**linical **E**xamination **S**kills (PACES). None of these variants has gained a world-wide acceptance and utilization as has the OSCE itself. Of the OSCE modifications the **P**ractical Assessment of **C**linical **E**xamination **S**kills (PACES) used mostly by the MRCP UK has received adoption by some other authorities such as the Faculty of Internal Medicine of the West African College of Physicians. Here we give only a short description of PACES, For interested readers, more detailed information may be obtained from the MRCP (UK) website.

10.2. OVERVIEW OF PACES

Practical **A**ssessment of **C**linical **E**xamination **S**kills (PACES) is the MRCP (UK) clinical examination that has been running since 2001. It is a modification of the popular OSCE system for examining medical postgraduates in Internal Medicine. It is partly structured with the scoring system being more of the global type rather than the checklist type of grading task components used in a typical OSCE. The following are some of the features of PACES.

Number of stations

There are typically five encounters or stations instead of OSCE's 15 – 25 stations. All stations are manned by examiners, there being no written stations. Each station lasts 20 minutes with a 5- minute interval in-between stations.

Examination Duration

Usually the whole circuit lasts 125 minutes, rather similar to standard OSCE's 120-150 minutes. There are no rest or written stations but the transition period of five minutes among stations more than makes up for a rest station/time for both candidates and examiners.

Station Tasks in PACES:

There may be more than one task at a given station but each task is given its own timing (by a local timer). Station 5 used to be more of a spot diagnosis or short cases of old. This multi-task station has been replaced by tasks on brief consultations in the UK examination. The Internal Medicine Faculty of the West African College of Physicians (FIMWACP) still uses the old system of four short encounters at Station 5. Like in OSCE, candidates go round the circuit manned by examiners. There are instructions to candidates, examiners, simulated and real patients on what should be done.

Instructions to Candidates and Examiners

These instructions are somewhat similar to those in OSCE but will usually include the candidate discussing with the examiners toward the end of the task session. Examiner /candidate interaction is more extensive than in a typical OSCE. For each station about 80% of the time is set outside for the candidate's performance under observation and reflection and the rest for discussion.

Scoring System:

Each examiner has a semi-structured marksheet to grade candidate performance but final grading is essentially global and subjective. The two examiners at each station score candidate performance using a guideline provided; they do not consult each other or harmonise marks as is often done in some traditional methods of examination. Thus each candidate will have 16 sets of marks from eight patients in the whole circuit.

Checklists or rating scales are not used in the PACES system in the manner they are used in OSCE. The assessment of each station is global in nature usually in the following categories: *Pass, Fail, and borderline*; or *Clear pass (CP), Borderline pass (BP), Borderline fail (BF), and Clear fail (CF)*. Modifications to the system are being made to infuse more objectivity in grading the candidate's performance.

Feedback forms

A feedback system is built into the examination for candidates who are unsuccessful at the examination.

OSCE Skills for Trainees in Medicine

Advantages and Limitations

The main advantages of PACES over the traditional long-short case assessment are that each candidate sees several patients and is assessed by at least 10 examiners. All the candidates encounter similar or same patients in eight or ten encounters. The examination like OSCE thus appears to be fair to the candidate.

The number of candidates interacting with a particular patient may be fewer than in OSCE but like in OSCE, patient fatigue can easily set in. The rather small number of stations in PACES may affect its reliability. The qualitative nature of the pass-fail decision process is associated with a high degree of subjectivity and is a major point of criticism of the PACES tool.

10.3. PACES STRUCTURE AND PROCEDURE

A PACES exercise consists of a circuit or carrousel of five stops, labelled stations 1, 2, 3, 4, and 5, see Figure 10.1. Stations 1 and 3 each have two substations, and Station 5 (now) has two substations in the MRCP (UK) examination but four in the FIMWACP examination.

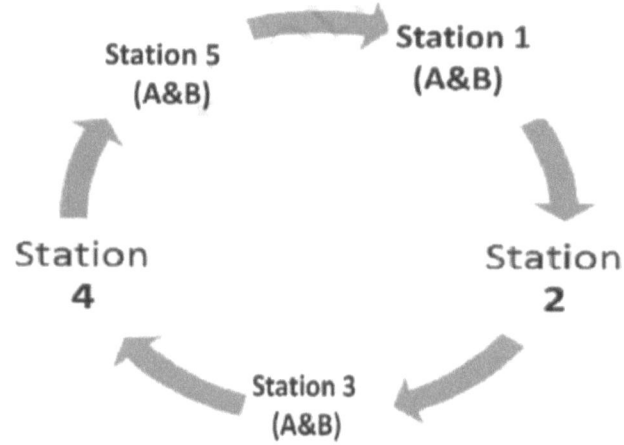

Figure 10.1. Schema of Practical Assessment of Clinical Examination Skills. *A PACES circuit consists of five main stations (stations 1-5), three (stations 1, 3, and 5) of which have substations. Each station is 'manned' by two clinical examiners. A time keeper directs movement of candidates among stations. Examiners or other assistants may help with 'local' timing within stations. *In current MRCP(UK) PACES, station 5 has two substations while in the Faculty of Internal Medicine of the West Africa College of Physicians the station has four substations.*

Each circuit takes five candidates at a time. Several circuits may be run simultaneously depending on the number of candidates, availability of examiners, and other resources. A candidate starts at one of the stations and moves in a clockwise direction on hearing the signal to do so as in OSCE. At each of stations 1, 3, and 5 there are two patients. A candidate spends a total of 10 minutes with each patient including the period of interaction with the examiners. At stations 2 and 4, there is one patient each (usually simulated patients) with whom the candidate have to interact for about 14 minutes, followed by about 5 minutes of interaction with the examiners (Table 10.1).

While each candidate spends a total of 20 minutes at each station, the management of station time varies from one station to another depending on the type of task at the station

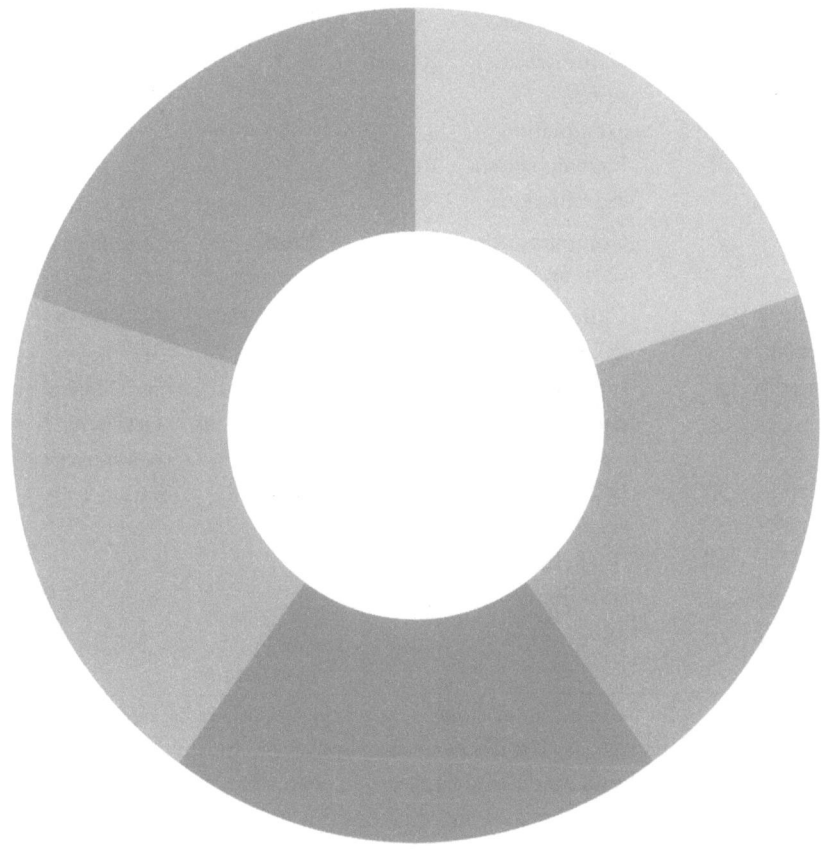

OSCE Skills for Trainees in Medicine

Table 10.1. PACES Structure and Activities

Event	Station	Theme	Duration	Activity	Position at first 20 min
Interval	1	History Taking	5 min	Read Instructions	Candidate 1 starts here,
*Start action	1A	Respiratory system examination	10 min	PE and Interaction with examiners	then moves to Station 2
	1B	Abdominal system examination	10 min		
Interval	2	History Taking	5 min	Read Instructions	Candidate 2 starts here,.
Start action	2	History Taking	20 min	PCI CEI	then moves to Station 3
Interval	3	Physical Examination	5 min	Read Instructions	Candidate 3 starts here
Start action	3A	Cardiovascular system examination	10 min	PCI	then moves to Station 4,.
	3B	Nervous system examination	10 min		
Interval	4	Communication skills and ethics	5 min	Read Instructions	Candidate 4 starts here,
Start action	4	Communication skills and ethics	20 min	PSI, CEI	then moves to Station 5
Interval	5	Integrated clinical assessment	5 min	Read Instructions	Candidate 5 starts here, then moves to Station 1
Start action	5A†	Brief clinical consultation 1	10 min	PCI, SEI	
	5B	Brief clinical consultation 2	10 min		
Interval	1	Physical Exam		Read Instructions	

* A candidate who starts at station 1 moves round the circuit and back to Station 1 where they end the exercise. The five candidates in each run move clockwise until all stations are covered by all candidates. †Station 5 has two substations in the current MRCP (UK) examination but four stations in the FIMWACP examination. *PCI, Patient- candidate interaction; CEI, Candidate –Examiner interaction*

What the Examiners are looking for in PACES?

Passing or failing a PACES station depends on the extent to which a candidate's performance meets the expectations of the examiners. The candidate's standing in the whole OSCE is the summation of your performance at each of the stations. The examiners are given the criteria for rating candidate station performance as satisfactory or otherwise. An examiner may score a candidate performance satisfactory or unsatisfactory. Sometimes the examiner may conclude that the candidate's performance is in the gray area of between satisfactory and unsatisfactory, not a pass but not quite a fail either. This is the *borderline performance* at a skill component. The examiner does this type of scoring for all the components of the task. For the candidate's overall performance rating for each encounter, the examiner scans his ratings for the subsets and then concludes on what they think of the candidate generally including aspects not on the checklist. They then score the candidate as follows:

- Clear pass with a score of 4 (satisfactory level 1)
- Borderline pass with a score of 3 (satisfactory pass level 2)
- Borderline fail with a score of 2 (unsatisfactory level 1)   and
- Clear fail with a score of 1 (unsatisfactory level 2)

10.4. COMPARISON OF OSCE AND PACES

PACES and OSCE have several similarities but also some important differences, as shown in Table 10.2. The main similarities are the use of several stations and examiners and the exposure of all candidates to same or similar clinical scenarios. On the other hand the major difference appears to be the scoring system: largely objective in OSCE but subjective in PACES. The OSCE also has room for assessment of more competencies besides purely clinical ones.

Table 10.2. Comparing PACES and OSCE

Characteristic	PACES	OSCE
Meaning of acronym	Practical Assessment of Clinical Examination Skills	Objective Structured Clinical Examination
Exam duration	About 2½ hours	Variable; range 1hour-3 hours
Number of stations	Five with three having substations	Varies from 8-30; some may be coupled
Duration of a station	20 min; but some time split between two or four tasks.	5-10 min for short stations but more time for long stations
Examiners/station	Two	One or two
Examiners per circuit	Minimum 10	Variable but usually not less than eight
Rest stations	None but has 5-min interval between stations	Average of one rest station to eight active stations
Written stations	None	Number variable; may be administered separately
Procedure stations	None	Often included
Veto stations	None	Sometimes included
Scoring system	Global using guidelines; but getting more objective	Various types including short answer questions
Standard setting	Partly criterion based	Reference or criterion based or combination
Main limitation	Subjective scoring	Short duration of stations
Main merit	Fairness, very clinical	Fairness, objective, clinical and practical skills assessed

Assessment of competencies appears to be more clinically oriented in PACES than in OSCE, as all stations have SPs or real patients. While all stations are manned by clinicians in PACES, in OSCE some stations are unmanned and yet others may be manned by non-physicians or SPs.

10.5. PACES CRITERIA FOR ASSESSING PERFORMANCE

The approaches to assessment of candidate's performance at each skill station are shown in Tables 10.3 – 10.6. The information contained therein is largely from the PACES website.

PACES

Assessing Performance at a PACES History-Taking Station

At the history- taking station (Station 2) the emphasis is on clinical communication skills; managing patient's concerns; ability to construct a sensible list of differential diagnosis, select proper management plan, and paying attention to the welfare and comfort of the patient. Table 10.3. shows how Station 2 is advisedly assessed.

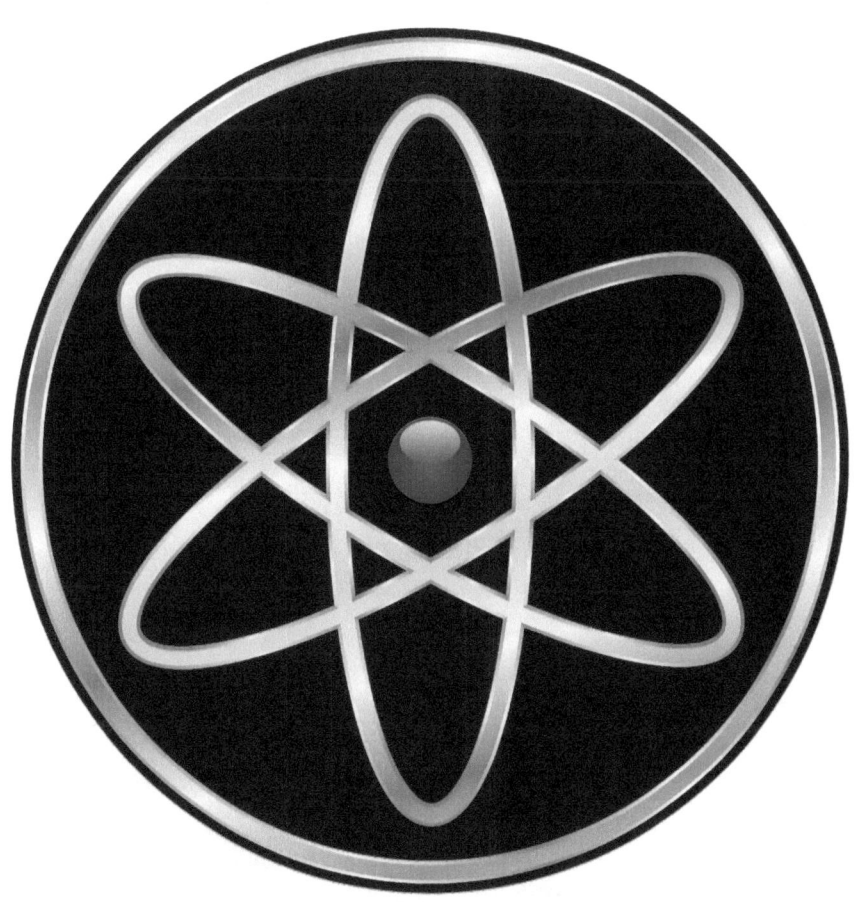

Table 10.3. Assessment Criteria for History Taking Skills in PACES

Satisfactory	BL	Unsatisfactory
Clinical Communications Skills		
• Elicits presenting complaint, reviews past, family and medication history, in a thorough, systematic, fluent and professional manner. • Assesses impact of symptoms on patient's occupation, lifestyle and activities of daily living. • Explains relevant clinical information in an accurate, clear, structured, comprehensive, fluent and professional manner.		• Omits important areas of the history, unsystematic • Appears unpractised and unprofessional, omits important information • Gives inaccurate information, uses jargon, poorly structured interview
Managing Patients' Concerns		
• Seeks, detects, acknowledges and attempts to address patient's concerns. • Confirms patient's knowledge and understanding, • Listens and is empathic		• Overlooks patient's concerns • Does not check knowledge and understanding • Poor listening, not empathic
Differential Diagnosis		
Constructs a sensible differential diagnosis, including the correct diagnosis		Poor differential diagnosis, fails to consider the correct diagnosis
Clinical Judgement		
Suggests a comprehensive, sensible and appropriate management plan		Unfamiliar with correct management plan, selects inappropriate management
Maintaining Patient Welfare		
Treats patient respectfully and sensitively and ensures his comfort, safety, and dignity		Causes patient physical or emotional discomfort, jeopardises patient safety

*BL, borderline performance

Assessing Communication Skills and Ethics (Station 4).

The communication skills and ethics station aims to assess the candidate's ability to guide and organize the interview with the subject (who may be a patient, relative, or surrogate, such as a healthcare worker), explain clinical information, apply clinical knowledge, including knowledge of ethics, to the management of the case or situation. The candidate is expected to provide emotional support and treat the patient with dignity and respect. Table 10.6. shows how Station 4 may be scored.

If the focus of the station is on ethics, the objectives to be scored may include one or more of the four basic ethical principles of autonomy, beneficence, nonmaleficence, and justice/equity i.e.

- Respecting the patient as a person; their medical best interests and wishes
- Using professional judgment;- in the face of uncertainty to communicate accurately and honestly
- Trying to do more good than harm
- Showing awareness of the principles of justice and equity

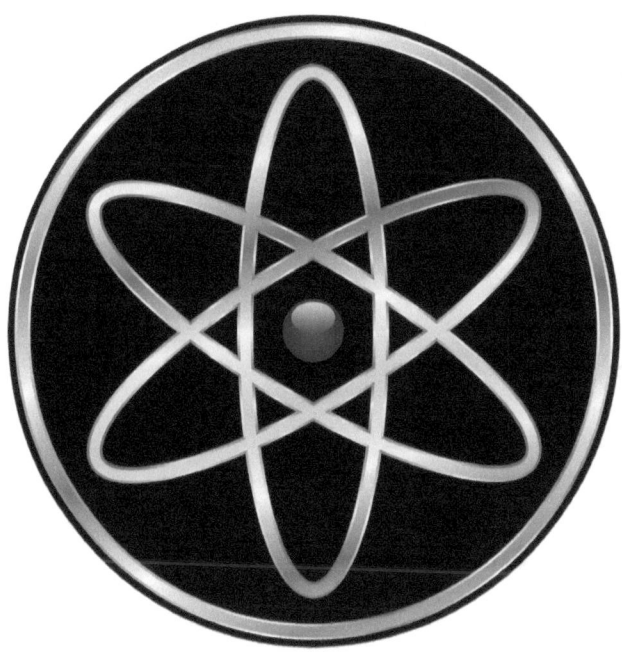

Table 10.4. Assessing Communication/Ethics Skills in PACES

Satisfactory	BL	Unsatisfactory

Clinical Communication Skills

Explains relevant clinical information in an accurate, clear, structured, comprehensive, fluent and professional manner		Omits important information; gives inaccurate or unclear information; poorly structured; uses jargon; appears unpractised and unprofessional

Managing Patient's Concerns

• Seeks, detects, acknowledges and attempts to address patient's or relative's concerns • Listens • Confirms patient's or relative's knowledge and understanding • Empathic		• Overlooks patient's or relative's concerns • Poor listening skills • Not empathic • Does not check knowledge and understanding

Clinical Judgement

• Suggests and/ or negotiates a sensible and appropriate management plan for the patient, relative or clinical situation • Can apply clinical knowledge, including knowledge of law and ethics, to this case		• Offers and/ or negotiates an inappropriate, incomplete or incorrect management plan • Cannot apply clinical knowledge, including knowledge of law and ethics, to this case

Maintaining Patient Welfare

Treats patient respectfully and sensitively and ensures comfort, safety and dignity		Causes patient physical or emotional discomfort; Jeopardises patient safety

*BL, borderline

Assessing Physical Examination Skills (at Stations 1, 3, ± 5)

At the **Physical Examination Skills (PES)** station the emphasis is on:
- demonstration of comprehensive and correct physical examination technique
- ability to detect physical signs (and not to 'manufacture physical signs')
- ability to construct a differential diagnosis

- ability to suggest sensible and appropriate treatment and investigation plans and
- being able to treat a patient with dignity and respect.

Table 10.5. shows s how a physical examination skills station is assessed.

Table 10.5. Assessment Criteria for Physical Exam Skills in PACES

Satisfactory	BL*	Unsatisfactory
Physical examination technique		
Correct, thorough, fluent, systematic and professional technique of inspection, palpation, percussion and auscultation		Incorrect techniques; Omits significant or important tests; unsystematic; hesitant and lacks confidence; unprofessional
Identifying Physical Signs		
Identifies correct physical signs; does not find signs that are not present		Misses important signs; finds signs that are not present
Differential Diagnosis		
Constructs a sensible differential diagnosis list including the correct diagnosis		Poor differential diagnosis; fails to consider the correct diagnosis
Clinical Judgement		
Suggests a sensible and appropriate management plan		Unfamiliar with correct management plan; offers inappropriate management
Maintaining Patient Welfare		
Treats patient respectfully and sensitively; ensures comfort, safety and dignity		Causes patient physical or emotional discomfort; jeopardises patient safety

*BL, borderline

Brief Clinical Consultation Skills

At the *Brief Clinical Consultation* skills station the emphasis is on demonstrating and integrating all the skills in the management of a patient who has been referred. The station aims to assess the way in which the candidate approaches a clinical problem in an integrated manner, using a combination of history taking, physical examination, and communication with a patient or a surrogate patient. Table 10.6 shows the criteria for assessing the *Brief Clinical Consultation Station*.

10.6. ATTRIBUTES OF A GOOD PERFORMANCE

The core skills (of communications/ethics, clinical judgement, management of patient's concerns, identification of physical sins, and maintenance of patient welfare), and the expected attributes of the good candidate at a PACES station would include the following qualities of a good clinician:

- *Communication Skills*
    - Defines purpose of interview
    - Avoids jargon
    - Uses open –ended and closed questions appropriately
    - Listens attentively
    - Reacts to cues
    - Negotiates
    - Empathises
    - Explains clearly
    - Summarises-confirms understanding
- *Clinical judgement/management*
    - Offers management plan that is comprehensive, sensible and appropriate
- *Managing Patient's Concerns*
    - Seeks, detects, acknowledges, attempts to address patient's concerns
    - Confirms patient's knowledge and understanding
    - Listens
    - Shows empathy

Table 10.6. Scoring Criteria for Brief Consultation

Satisfactory	BL*	Unsatisfactory
Clinical Communications Skills		
Elicits history relevant to the complaint and explains information to the patient in a focused, fluent and professional manner		Omits important areas of the history; unpractised; unprofessional; poor explanation to the patient
Physical Examination		
Correct; Appropriate; Practised; and Professional		Incorrect techniques; omits significant or important tests; inappropriate focus to examination; hesitant and lacks confidence; unprofessional
Clinical Judgement		
Selects a comprehensive, sensible and appropriate management plan		Unfamiliar with correct management plan; selects inappropriate management
Managing Patient's Concerns		
Seeks, detects, acknowledges and attempts to address patient's concerns; confirms patient's knowledge and understanding; listens; and is empathic		Overlooks patient's concerns; poor listening; not empathic; and does not check knowledge and understanding
Identifying Physical Signs		
Identifies correct physical signs; does not find signs that are not present		Misses important physical signs; finds signs that are not present
Differential Diagnosis		
Constructs a sensible differential diagnosis list, including the correct diagnosis		Poor differential diagnosis; fails to consider the correct diagnosis
Clinical Judgement		
Proposes a comprehensive, sensible and appropriate management plan		Unfamiliar with correct management plan; selects inappropriate management
Maintaining Patient Welfare		
Treats patient respectfully and sensitively and ensures comfort, safety, and dignity		Causes patient physical or emotional discomfort; jeopardises patient safety

*BL, borderline

- **Identifying Physical Signs**
  - Exhibits correctness of technique
  - Is thorough, fluent and systematic
  - Shows professional technique of examination (palpation, percussion and auscultation)
  - Identifies correct physical signs
  - Does not find signs that are not present
- ***Differential Diagnosis***
  Constructs a sensible differential diagnosis list that includes the correct diagnosis
- ***Ethical Principles***
  - Respects the patient as a person, their medical best interests and their wishes
  - Uses professional judgment to communicate accurately and honestly
  - Tries to do more good than harm
  - Shows awareness of the principles of justice and equity
- ***Maintaining Patient Welfare***

Treats patient respectfully and sensitively and ensures comfort, safety and dignity

10.7. ADVICE FOR THE PACES CANDIDATE

1. The PACES system is heavily clinical and you must therefore up your clinical skills from history taking to patient management. Be familiar with the nature of all five stations. Read a clinical methods book and revise your applied physiology
2. Practise and perfect your history-taking skills repeatedly on all systems. Make a list of common symptoms and create a checklist for each.
3. Practise generously on how to examine the different systems or regions of the body (especially abdomen, cardiovascular system, respiratory system, and the nervous system).
4. Learn and master good methods of communication especially teaching patients, explaining to patients and breaking bad news
5. Be sure of your physical findings and their possible meaning

6. It is bad to omit important physical findings; it is a "crime" and unethical to claim to find or manufacture signs that are not present.
7. Know what signs to look for in particular conditions and be clear of the causes of such findings.
8. Have perfected your chosen approach of presenting your findings from the history and/or physical examinations
9. In presenting your findings, give both the positive findings and relevant negative findings
10. You must be able to interpret the physical findings and situate them in the context of the diagnosis in the index patient or case
11. When required to make a diagnosis, make a *complete diagnosis* and justify your diagnosis based on your findings in the patient before you.
12. In preparation for your clinical examinations be they OSCE or PACES, get used to a method of making a rapid diagnosis: Use either the *pattern recognition* approach or the *hypothetico-deductive* method.
13. Plan your investigation and management before presentation. Have a reliable method of planning.
14. Base your diagnosis on the findings present in the patient you examined, not on the textbook features to be found in that condition.
15. Make your investigation and treatment plans relevant to the patient before you or on whom you have just examined; not just a general approach.
16. Know the common cases and scenarios (and their causes) that occur in local practice and in PG examinations
17. In planning management use the **SOAP** approach: list the problems, for each determine what tests to be done and what treatment including referral should be done.

10.8. CHAPTER TEN SUMMARY

- PACES is the MRCP (UK) modification of OSCE for the assessment of clinical skills of postgraduate trainees in Internal Medicine.

- A PACES circuit consists of eight or 10 manned encounters at five stations.
- There are no written or unmanned stations in PACES unlike OSCE.
- The whole circuit of PACES lasts 125 minutes.
- Each station is manned by two clinical examiners.
- Scoring is largely global although the basis for pass or failure is stated.
- The merits of PACES include its usage of same and several examiners and clinical scenarios to test every candidate.
- The scoring system appears to be evolving from subjectivity to some degree of objectivity as in OSCE.

10.9. CHAPTER 10 RECAP EXERCISES

1. What does the acronym PACES mean?
2. How many stations are usually there in a PACES circuit?
3. List the stations and their descriptions or titles.
4. How long does a full PACES *station* last?
5. What skills are the examiners looking for at
   a. the physical examination skills station?
   b. the communications skills station?
   c. ethics station
6. What are the attributes of a poor or unsatisfactory performance at a history station?

10.10 BIBLIOGRAPHY AND RESOURCES, page 249

Glossary of Medical Education Terms

Ability. The level of successful performance of the objects of measurement on a variable.

Achievement test. A test designed to measure and quantify a person's knowledge and/or skill.

Action term. A verb used to describe desired objectives or outcomes

Assessment. The process of measuring an individual's progress and accomplishments against defined standards and criteria.

Attitude. (a) The emotions or feelings that influence a learner's desire or choice to perform a particular task. (b) A positive alteration in personal and professional beliefs, values, and feelings that will enable the learner to use skills and knowledge to implement positive change in the work environment.

Behaviour. An overt or covert activity that is capable of being measured.

Blueprint. A template used to define the content of a given test. In medical education, it is often designed as a matrix or a series of matrices.

Borderline methods (of standard setting). A method of determining the pass mark in performance tests

Case-based discussion (CbD). An assessment, in which the trainee chooses case records from recently seen patients in whose notes they have made entries. The assessor will then select one of these for a case-based discussion. This process assesses clinical decision-making and medical knowledge in the care of the trainee's patients and enables the assessor to assess the reasons for the trainee's actions and choices.

Checklists. Evaluation instruments where categories are checked off (e.g., done/not done).

Compare and contrast. Provide a description of similarities and differences (eg. table form)

Competency. The knowledge, skill, attitude or combination of these, that enables one to effectively perform the activities of a particular occupation or role to the standards expected. Compare this with performance which denotes what someone is actually doing in a real life situation.

Cognition. The mental or intellectual activity or process of possessing intellectual skill or knowledge.

Criterion. (a) The standard by which something is measured. (b) In the validation of test and measurement instruments, the standard against which test instruments are correlated to indicate the accuracy with which they predict human performance in some specified area.

Criterion referencing (assessment). Measures performance against an absolute standard, i.e. each trainee's performance is matched against a benchmark (usually the pass mark). In contrast norm referencing ranks each student's performance against all the others in the same cohort, with a (usually) predetermined number of the top students passing.

Critically evaluate. Appraise the evidence available to support the hypothesis; give the pros and cons

Curriculum. An educational plan that spells out what goals and objectives should be achieved, what topics should be covered and what methods are to be used for learning, teaching and assessment.

Curriculum standards describe skills, knowledge, attitudes and values, what teachers are supposed to teach and what students are expected to learn.

Diagnostic or Formative Test. Instruments used to determine attainment of supporting skills and knowledge necessary to perform the terminal objectives. Diagnostic tests are used during formative evaluation of the instructional system to predict student success, and to identify and correct weaknesses in the instruction.

Direct observation of procedural skills (DOPS). An assessment in which the trainees are observed with real patients and are assessed and provided with feedback on procedural skills. It is similar to mini-CEX in both of which feedback is given by the assessor immediately after the assessment.

Discriminator. An item that separates well between weak and strong test candidates, stronger trainees performing statistically better than weaker ones.

Domain. The scope of knowledge, skills, competencies and professional characteristics that can be combined for practical reasons into one cluster.

Evaluation. The process of determining the quality and value of an educational programme and/or the assessment of individuals on the programme. Generally 'assessment' is used of individuals and 'evaluation' of programmes.

Examination. A formal, controlled method or procedure to assess an individual's knowledge, skills and abilities. Examinations might involve written or oral responses, or observation of the trainee performing practical tasks.

Examination Blueprint. A matrix that relates the knowledge, skills, and attitude areas that are being assessed to the questions or stations which were designed to accomplish this task.

Feedback. A process by which a teacher provides information to the learners about their performance for the purpose of improvement.

Fail. Awarded a score below the pass mark.

Formative assessment is a test that does not contribute to final pass/fail decisions. It is carried out for the purpose of improvement rather than pass/fail decision making. This assessment informs trainers and learners about strengths, weaknesses and any problem areas.

Goal. A general aim towards which to strive.

Hypothetico-deductive method of making a diagnosis; start by developing hypotheses to explain a patient's clinical features and apply collected data to test a hypothesis in order to try and confirm or exclude a diagnosis. Students should start with this method; compare pattern recognition of diagnosis.

Knowledge. The acquisition or awareness of facts, data, information, ideas or principles to which one has access through formal or individual study, research, observation experience, and/or intuition. Unlike performance, knowledge is not directly observable.

Learning. A change in behaviour of the trainee or learner as a result of experience.

Learning outcomes. The consequences expected for training for each of the areas of practice.

List. Provide a list, itemize, enumerate

Listening skills. Ability to listen to patients, tolerating their negative affect; hearing and acting upon constructive criticism; and not dominating discussion at the expense of discussant.

Metrics. Measurement tools such as test and measurement instruments used for assessing the progress of trainees with respect to the standards specified for instructional system development.

Management, of medical disorders, proper evaluation, investigations and treatment

Mini-Clinical Evaluation Exercise (mini-CEX). Mini-CEX is a brief observation of a trainee's interaction with a patient. It aims to assess the clinical skills, attitudes, and behaviours required for providing a high standard of patient care. Feedback is provided immediately after by the assessor and trainees are able to identify strengths and areas for improvement.

Mnemonics. Learning aids or aid memoires organized in the form of a word or a phrase (e.g., SOCRATES for history taking).

Models, Mannequins and Simulators are used to facilitate demonstrations and hands-on clinical learning. Famous mannequins include *Resusci Annie* which is used for instructions in cardio-pulmonary resuscitation and Harvey (an electronic heart machine that permits the simulation of a variety of diagnostic and therapeutic interventions).

Most likely. Give the single (one) most likely answer

Multiple choice. An item where the trainee selects what they consider to be the correct answer from a list of options. Commonly used in MCQs (multiple choice questions) and EMQs (extended matching questions).

Multiple choice question (MCQ). A lead-in statement followed by a homologous list of four or five options from which the candidate selects the best answer, in the single best answer system.

Norm referencing. A method of establishing passing and failing trainees based on their performance in relation to each other, rather than to an established standard (criterion referencing).

Objective (noun). A statement that specifies precisely what learning behaviour is to be exhibited by the student, the given conditions under which the behaviour will be accomplished in the instructional system, and the minimum standards of learner performance required to demonstrate mastery of the objective.

Objective (adjective). Factual, not influenced by personal views or bias.

OSCE. Objective Structured Clinical Examination - a multi-station clinical examination (typically having 15 to 25 stations). Candidates spend a designated time (usually 5 to 10 minutes) at each station demonstrating a clinical skill or competency at each. Stations frequently feature real or (more often) simulated patients. Artefacts such as radiographs, lab reports and photographs are also commonly used.

OSLER. Objective Structured Long Case Examination Record. A clinical assessment that consists of 10 items, (four on history, three on physical examination and three on management and clinical insight). It is based on a candidate taking a formal history and completing an examination on a patient. The suggested time for the OSLER examination is 30 minutes.

Outline. Provide a summary of the important points

PACES. See Practical Assessment of Examination Skills

Pass. To achieve a score (mark) that allows progress in training or successful completion of an examination. A pass mark is the score that allows a trainee to pass an assessment.

Pattern recognition approach to diagnosis. A diagnosis based on experience, symptoms and signs; used by experts or experienced clinicians; matching the patients disease features to an appropriate illness picture.

Performance. The application of competence in real life; denotes what a student or clinician actually does in their encounter with patients, their relatives and carers, colleagues, team members and other members of staff, etc. *Performance* describes the observable candidate behaviour (or the product of that behaviour) that is acceptable to the instructor as proof that the student has accomplished a learning behaviour to an acceptable standard of completeness or accuracy, and that learning has occurred. It contrasts with cognitive or knowledge assessment.

Post-test. A test designed to measure student performance on objectives taught during a unit of instruction; used after exposure to an instructional programme to measure the changes that have occurred during instruction.

Practical Assessment of Examination Skills (PACES). A circuit of performance based on clinical encounters used for assessment of postgraduates by MRCP (UK). It consists of five stations, each manned by two examiners and lasts 20 minutes.

Pre-test. A test designed to measure student performance on objectives to be taught during a unit of instruction and student performance on entry into the course of instruction. Used to measure the student's ability to attain intended each objective of a course.

Professionalism. Adherence to a set of values comprising statutory professional obligations, formally agreed codes of conduct and the informal expectations of patients and colleagues. Key professional values include acting in the patients' best interest and maintaining the standards of competence and knowledge expected of members of highly trained professions. These standards include ethical elements such as integrity, probity, accountability, duty and honour. In addition to medical knowledge and skills, medical professionals should present psychosocial and humanistic qualities such as caring, empathy, and humility.

Quality assurance. A system of procedures, checks or audits that evaluates and monitors the work and the products of an institute, and proposes corrective measures, if necessary, to ensure that the outcomes are met as anticipated.

Rating scale. A scale used to measure trainee ability.

Raw score. A test mark that has not been modified.

Reliability. The degree to which a test and measurement instrument can be expected to yield the same result upon repeated administration to the same population. It is an expression of the consistency and reproducibility (precision) of measurements and is usually expressed as a reliability coefficient (r), which should be a value between 1 and 0.

Result. The outcome of a test.

Round robin. A training method in which the trainees play different roles in turn e.g. as student, then as examiner, then as a patient.

Rubric. A point on a rating scale representing a discrete level of candidate ability. An important characteristic of a rubric is that it is defined by a descriptor, explaining the level of ability that the rating scale point is related to.

Score. The mark obtained by a candidate in a test.

Self-assessment. A process of evaluation of one's own achievements, behaviour, professional performance and competencies. Self-assessment is an important part of self-directed and life-long learning.

Short answer question. A question that requires the trainee to construct and write down an appropriate answer briefly; i.e. a word, a sentence, a paragraph or two-three paragraphs.

Simulated patients. Individuals such actors who are not ill but adopt a patient's history or physical signs and role for learning or assessment in medical education. Simulated patients can also be individuals from the community or other health care providers. SPs are particularly useful in performance-based assessment such as OSCE. Also referred to as standardised patient.

Single best answer (SBA) questions. The term used in tests for one-from-five MCQs.

Skill. The ability to perform a job-related activity that contributes to the effective performance of an entire task. Skills involve physical or manipulative activities that require intellectual skills (knowledge) for their execution, and that also have specific requirements for speed, accuracy, or coordination. **Skill is** usually gained by training or experience.

SOAP approach, a method of keeping patient's records as part of the problem oriented medical records system; **S** stands for subjective findings; **O** stands for objective findings; **A** stands for Assessment, and **P** stands for Plan.

Standard. A criterion, gauge, yardstick or touchstone by which judgments or decisions may be made.

Standard setting. The process of establishing a cut point for passing or failing candidates
at a summative assessment.

Standardised patients. These are individuals who have been trained to reliably reproduce the history and/or physical findings of a particular case. They can be real patients who have been "standardized" for the purpose of education or they can be *simulated patients* who are actors trained to reliably reproduce clinical histories and physical signs.

Structured Standardised Oral Examination. An oral examination based on predetermined clinical scenarios, carefully selected and developed by experienced clinician examiners to represent the outcomes; assessed and marked by trained examiners using structured, pre-validated rating scale rubrics with anchored descriptors; purpose of the tool is to ensure that all the examinees receive a similar form of assessment, in terms of content, outcomes, item difficulty and examiner leniency.

Summative assessment is a test that occurs at the end of a course primarily to provide information about whether or not the student has reached the required standard and is used to take pass/fail decisions.

Syllabus. A list, or some other kind of summary description, of course contents or topics that might be tested in examinations. It is a shorter version of the detailed curriculum.

Test. A set of questions or exercises measuring knowledge, skills, attitudes and/or professionalism.

Triangulation. The principle - particularly important in workplace based assessment - that whenever possible, evidence of progress, attainment or difficulties should be obtained from more than one source, on more than one occasion and, if possible, using more than one assessment method.

True-false item examination. A written examination with a series of statements that the candidate/trainee has to identify either as 'true' or 'false'.

True/False MCQs. A lead-in statement followed by a list of four or five options all of which may be true or false; the candidate is required to identify the true and false answers.

True score. A trainee's score on a test without measurement error - true score is the observed score minus the error.

Validity. In the realm of assessment, validity refers to the degree to which a measurement instrument truly measures what it is supposed to measure. It is concerned with whether the right things are being assessed, in the right way, and with a positive influence of learning.

Viva voce. A traditional form of oral exam, where one or more examiners ask random questions at the candidate in a face-to-face interview or discussion. Each candidate may receive a different exam with regard to the examiners, assessment content, assessment outcomes, item difficulty and examiner leniency. In a structured viva voce, candidates receive similar questions and are scored in a similar structured manner.

Weighting. Assigning different values or scores to different items, reflecting, for example, their importance or difficulty in order to increase the effectiveness of a test.

Workplace Based Assessment (WBA). A workplace-based assessment measures what doctors actually do in practice; evaluating a range of competencies that a trainee uses during day-to-day encounters with patients.

Written Examination. Written examinations are typically characterised by supervision and time- restriction for completion. The question types include Multiple choice questions (MCQs); True/false (T/F) questions; matching items and short answer or structured response questions; and extended answers or essays. Written examinations test mostly cognition and contrasts with performance-based assessments such as OSCE.

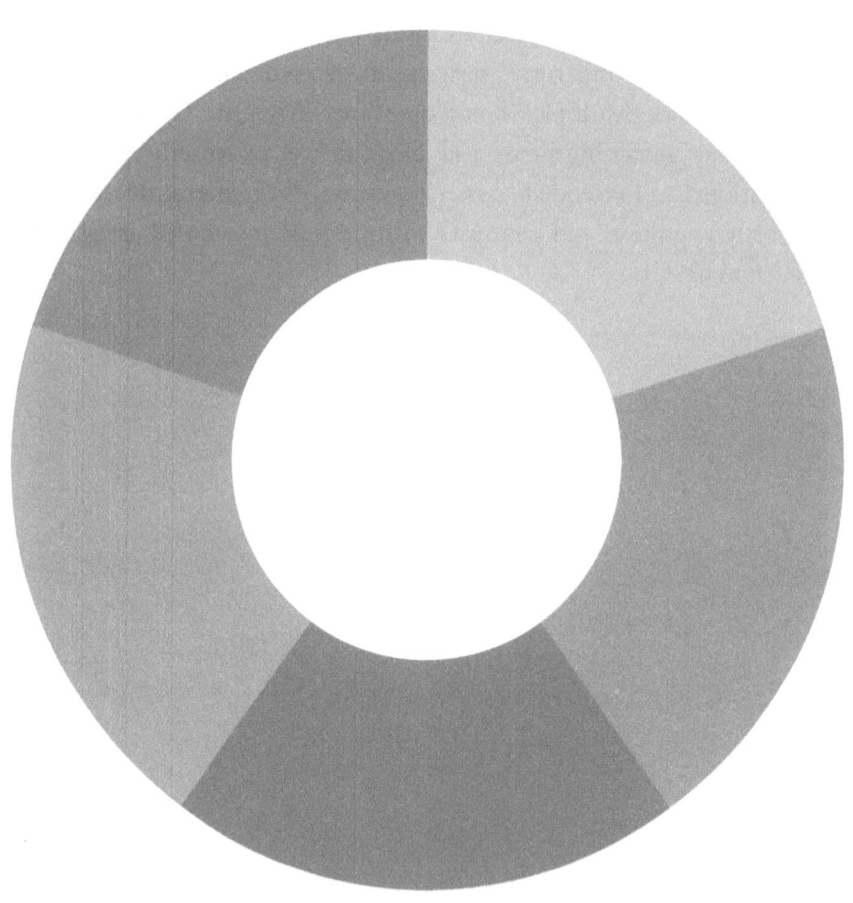

Bibliography and Resources

Chapter 1. Assessment of Trainee Performance in Medicine
Bloom B. S. (1956). *Taxonomy of Educational Objectives, Handbook I: The Cognitive Domain.* New York: David McKay Co Inc.

FAIMER (n.d.). International medical education directory. Retrieved 30 January 2008, from http://imed.ecfmg.org/

Miller G. The assessment of clinical skills/competence/performance. Acad Med 1990;65:S63–S67.

Chapter 2. Overview of Objective Structured Clinical Examination
Cushieri A, Gleeson F A, Harden R M, et al. A new approach to a final examination in surgery, use of the objective structured clinical examination. Ann Royal College of Surgeons of England 1979; 61: 400–405

Dhamija B, Green M. Student Succeeding in your OSCE BMJ 2012;20:e1656X

Sloan DA, Donnelly MB, Johnson SB, et al. Use of an Objective Structured Clinical Examination (OSCE) to measure improvement in clinical competence during the surgical internship. Surgery; 1993; 114: 343–50.

Tervo RC, Dimitrievich E, Trujillo AL, *et al.* The Objective Structured Clinical Examination (OSCE) in the clinical clerkship: an overview. S D J Med. 1997; 50:153-6.

Chapter 3. History - Taking Skills Station
Exam formats/136_e.php], Accessed February 18, 2010.
Format of the Comprehensive Objective Examination in Internal

http://docstig.isgreat.org/year5.html: extensive notes, examples
http://www.nhs.uk/video/pages/medialibrary.aspx?Tag=Children+and+babies+&Page=4
http://www.nhs.uk/video/pages/medialibrary.aspx?Tag=Children+and+babies+&Page=4
Medicine. 2009 [http://rcpsc.medical.org/residency/certification/
Swanson DB, Clauser BC, Case SM. Clinical skills assessment with standardized patients in high-stakes tests: a framework for thinking about score precision, equating and security. Adv Health Sci Educ 1999; 4:67-106.

Chapter 4. Communication Skills and Ethics Station

A model for communication skills assessment across the undergraduate curriculum.
Accreditation Council for Graduate Medical Education. ACGME Outcome Project. Retrieved Jun 5, 2005 from www.acgme.org/Outcomes).
Beale EA, Kudelka AP. SPIKES—a six-step protocol for delivering bad news: application to the patient with cancer. Oncologist 2000;5:302–311.
Dennis BD, Dwinnell B, Platt F. Invite, Listen, and Summarize: A Patient-Centered Communication Technique Acad Med. 2005; 80:29-32.
Emery B, Klamm K. Effective Listening in D.F. Beer (editor) Writing and Speaking in the Technology Professions. A Selected reprint volume, IEEE Professional Communication Society, IEEE Press 1992. New York: 255-257
Haynes ME. Becoming an Effective Listener in D.F. Beer (editor) Writing and Speaking in the Technology Professions. A Selected reprint volume, IEEE Professional Communication Society, IEEE Press 1992. New York: 251-254
Hobgood C, Harward D, Newton K, et al. The Educational Intervention "GRIEV-ING". http://classroomclipart.com/clipart/page-72/Clipart/Facial_Expressions.html
http://nyumacy.med.nyu.edu/
http://www.acgme.org/outcome/assess/IandC_Index.asp
Makoul G. Essential elements of communication in medical encounters: the Kalamazoo consensus statement. Acad Med. 2001;76:390–393.

Rider EA, Hinrichs MM, Lown BA. Teaching communication in clinical clerkships: models from the **Macy Initiative** in Health Communications. Med Teach. 2006;28:e127-34. http://depts.washington.edu/bioethx/topics/badnws.html http://www.aafp.org/afp/20011215/1975.pdf
www.iht.com/articles/2006/01/11/healthscience/sncancer.php
www.mja.com.au/public/issues/171_6_200999/maguire/maguire.html
www.postgradmed.com/issues/2002/09_02/editorial_sep.htm

Chapter 5. Physical Examination Skills Station

McMaster University Program for Educational Development. (1995) *Evaluation Methods: A Resource Handbook.* (Shannon S, Norman G, Eds.) Hamilton ON: McMaster University, p.71.

Nayer M. An Overview of the Objective Structured Clinical Examination. Physiotherapy Canada. 1993; 45: 171-178

Newbie DI, Swanson DB. Psychometric characteristics of the objective structured clinical examination. Medical Education. 1988;22: 325-334

Stratford PW, Thomson MA, Sanford J, *et al.* Effect of Station Examination Item Sampling on Generalizability of Student Performance. Physical Therapy 1990; 70: 31-36.

Walker HK, Hall WD, Hurst JW, editors. Clinical Methods: The History, Physical, and Laboratory Examinations. 3rd edition. Boston: Butterworths; 1990.

Chapter 6. Practical Procedure Skills Station

Berg RA, Hemphill R, Abella BS, *et al.* Part 5: Adult Basic Life Support. 2010 American Heart Association Guidelines for Cardiopulmonary Resuscitation and Emergency Cardiovascular Care. Supplement to Circulation. 2010; 122: S685-705

http://circ.ahajournals.org/content/vol122/18_suppl_3.toc

Hupfl M, Selig HF, Naggle P, *et al.* Chest-compression-only versus standard cardiopulmonary resuscitation: a meta-analysis. The Lancet. 2010; 376: 1552-7

Newble D, Cannon R. *A Handbook for Medical Teachers*, 3rd edn. London: Kluwer Academic Publishers, 1994

Pickering TG, Hall JE, Appel LJ, *et al.* Recommendations for blood pressure measurement in humans and experimental animals: Part 1: blood pressure measurement in humans: a statement for professionals from the Subcommittee of Professional and Public Education of the AHA Council on HBP. Circulation 2005; 111:697-716.

Sayre MR, Koster RW, Botha M, *et al.* Adult Basic Life Support: 2010 International Consensus on Cardiopulmonary Resuscitation and Emergency cardiovascular Care Science with Treatment Recommendations. Circulation. 122 (16 Suppl 2): S298-41

Chapter 7. Objective Structured Practical Examination

Ananthakrishnan N. Objective structured clinical/practical Examination (OSCE/OSPE). JPGM 1993;3:82-4.

Editorial: A brief overview regarding various aspects of Objective Structured Practical Examination (OSPE): Pak J Physiol 2007;3: 234-8

Harden RM, Gleeson FA. Assessment of clinical competencies using an objective structured clinical examination (OSCE) In: ASME Medical Education Booklet No. 8. Dundee: ASME; 1979.

http://www.pps.org.pk/58 PJP/5-1/Hasan.pdf

Patil NG, Saing H. Wong J. Role of OSCE in Evaluation of Practical Skills. An International Journal of Education in Practice for Educators in the Health Sciences, 2003;25: 12-16

Chapter 8. The OSCE Written Station

http://www.newmediamedicine.com/forum/search.php?searchid=3215888

Siddiqui A. Objective Structured Clinical Examination: a valid and reliable assessor of clinical competency. International Journal of Students' Research, North America, 1, jun. 2011. Available at: http://www.ijsronline.com/index.php/IJSR/article/view/80/253>. Date accessed: 06 Apr. 2012.

Chapter 9. The Structured Oral Examination Station

Anastakis DJ, Cohen R, Reznick RK. The structured oral examination as a method for assessing surgical residents. Am J Surg. 1991;162:67-70.

Daelmans HEM, Albert JJA, Scherpbier C, et al. Reliability of clinical oral examinations re-examined Medical Teacher 2001;23: 422-424

Davis MH, Ponnamperuma G, McAleer S, *et al*. Examiners' Manual. Joint Committee on Intercollegiate Examinations. ISBN: 1-871749-08-5

http://informahealthcare.com/doi/abs/10.1080/01421590126522

http://www.surgeons.org/media/384427/GDL_May2011_Urology_ Fellowship _Examination_Notes_to_Candidates.pdf

Kelly SP, Weiner SG, Anderson PD, *et al*. Learner perception of oral and written examinations in an international medical training program Int J Emerg Med. 2010; 3: 21–26.

Kshirsagar SV, Fulari SP. Structured Oral Examination – Student's perspective Anatomica Karnataka, 2011; 5: 28-31

Wiggins MN, Harper RA. Implementing a Structured Oral Examination into a Residency Program: Getting Started. Ophthalmic Surgery, Lasers & Imaging 2008; 39: 40-48

www.surgeons.org/.../GDL_May2011_Urology_Fellowship_Examination

Chapter 10. Practical Assessment of Clinical Examination Skills

Anon. PACES: practical assessment of clinical examination skills. The new MRCP(UK) clinical examination. J R Coll Physicians Lond 2000;34:57–60.

Bessant R, Bessant D, Chesser A, *et al*. Analysis of predictors of success in the MRCP (UK) PACES examination in candidates attending a revision course. Postgrad Med J 2006;82:145–149. doi: 10.1136/pmj.2005.035998

Dacre J, Besser M, White P; MRCP(UK) PART 2 Clinical Examination (PACES): a review of the first four examination sessions (June 2001 - July 2002). Clin Med. 2003;3:452-9.

http://www.e-paces.com/

http://www.mrcpuk.org/paces/pages/pacesformat.aspx

http://www.mrcpuk.org/SiteCollectionDocuments/PACES-candidate-guidenotes.pdf

http://www.rxpgonline.com/article1346.html http://www.mrcpuk.org/PACES/Pages/_Home.aspx

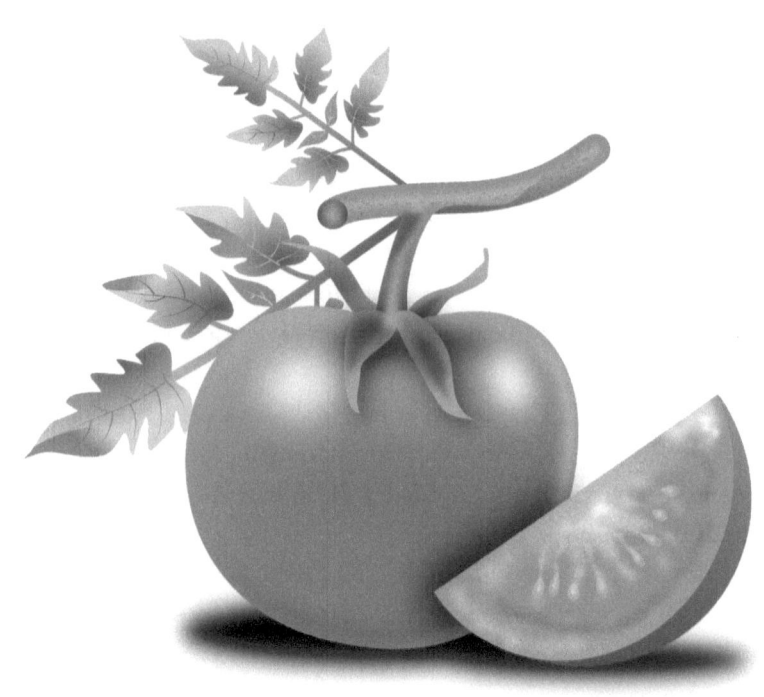

INDEX

ABCDE, model for breaking bad news, **68**
Abdominal pain
    examination skills of, **108** ff
    taking history of, **40,** *Table 2.1*
Abdominal examination skills, assessment of, **110 ff**
Advice to candidates on
    handling oral examination , **212**
    handling PACES stations, **234**
    practical procedure station, **141**
Alcoholism, interviewing skills about, **88**
Algorithm, for basic life support, **156**
American Heart Association, protocol for basic life support, **158**
Analysis, biochemical, at an OSPE station, **170**
Analytic experiment, scoring of, **171,** *Table 7.2*
Appearance of person , role in communication, **62**
Ask-talk-ask, method of patient education, **81**
Assessable competencies at
    history taking station , **38**
    physical examination station, **95**
    structured viva station , **201**
    written station, **181**
Assessment of history-taking skills, guide for, **40**

Assessment, of trainees
    benefits to stakeholders, **1**
    definition and purpose of, **1**
    tools for, **5**
Assessment for learning, purpose of, **5.** *See also formative assessment*
Assessment of learning, purpose of, **5.** *See also summative assessment*
Assessment tools, appropriate for competencies, **7,** *Table 1.2*
Autonomy, ethical principle of, **60**

Basic life support, algorithm for, **158**
Basic life support skills
    in hospital setting, **151**
    outside hospital setting, **158**
Beneficence, ethical principle of, **60**
Blood pressure
    measurement skills, rating scale for, **144** *Table 6.1*
    checklist for skills assessment , **174,** *Table 7.3*
Blood transfusion skills, rating of, **156**
Bloom, domains of educational activities of, **2**
Borderline performance rating, at PACES stations, **223**
Breaking bad news
    assessment of skills for , **74,** *Table 4.3*
    protocols for , **68**

rating objectives, **74ff**
postgraduate level, **74**
undergraduate level, **75**
Breathlessness, history-taking of, **53**

CAGE, in assessment of alcoholism, **88**
Candidate instructions at
communication station, **66, passim**
history taking station, **32, passim**
physical examination station, **96. passim**
Structured oral examination station, **204, passim**
Cannula insertion, assessing skills of, **182**
Cardiovascular system, examination skills of, **119**
Checklist as a tool for
assessment of candidates, **21**
use in assessment of procedure skills, **174**
Circuit, schematic depiction of
Objective Structured Clinical Examination, **11** *Figure 2.1*
Objective Structured Practical Examination, **116,** *Figure 7.1*
Practical Assessment of Clinical Examination Skills, **224,** *Figure 10.1*
Clinical communication, core skills for, **64**
Clinical communication skills, major categories of, **61**
Clinical performance in PACES, of candidates
assessing of, at communication station, **232**

assessing of, at physical examination station, **233**
at history-taking station, **230**
criteria for assessment of, **228**
Communication and ethics station
candidate instructions at, **66, passim**
features of, **66**
materials and equipment at, **66**
Communication skills
assessment models for, **68**
assessment of, **69**
essential, for health care providers, 68
required steps in processing information, **64**
Communication, types of, **64f**
Competencies
clinical, frequently assessed, **2**
examinable, at a written station, **181**
expected of trainees, **18, passim**
Cognition, Bloom's levels of, **6,** *Table 1.1*
Communication skills, assessment criteria for, 218, *Table 10.4*
Communication, basic steps in, **64,** *Table 4.1*
Comparison, of OSCE and PACES, **228**, *Table 10.1*
Competency question, at Structured *Viva*, **202**
Consensus, on essential communication skills, **62**
Consent, skills at obtaining of, **91**
Consultation, assessment criteria, in PACES, **235**, *Table 10.6*
Couplet station in OSCE, **18**

INDEX

Death certification, assessment of, how to, **155**
Default question, at Structured Viva, **202**
Depression, history taking skills on, **56**
Descriptors, of performance, at physical examination, **115**
Diagnosis, explanation of, to patient, **84**
Diagnostics, for physical examination station, **98**
Dimensions, of a symptom in history taking, **34**
Discharging patient home, station objectives for, **86**
Do's and Don'ts, at history taking, **43**
Domains, cognitive, of Bloom's, **3**
Dress code, for candidates in OSCE, **25**

Ectopic pregnancy, abdominal pain due to, history taking in, **51**
Effective listening, how to, **78**
Elderly patient discharging home, station objectives for, **86**
Electrocardiogram, at a station, **190** *Figure 8.4*
Emotions, facial expression showing, **63**, *Figure 4.2*
Empathy
 facial expression, depicting, **63ff**
 how to show, **78**
Escape question, use in structured viva, **202**
Ethical principles, types of, **60, 230**
Ethics, medical, main principles of, **60**
Examinable themes, potentials, amples for OSPE, **178**
Examiner's expectations of candidate
 at a communication station, **69**
 at a history station, **33**
 at a physical examination station, **99**
 of performance in OSCE, **18**
 of performance in PACES, **227**
Examiner, information for,
 at a communication station, **64**
 at a history taking station **91**
 at a physical examination station, **101**
 at a structured *viva* station, **205ff**
 in OSCE, **18f**
 in PACES, **223**
Examples of
 communication stations, **71ff**
 history taking stations, **47ff**
 physical examination stations, **115ff**
 practical procedure stations, **151ff**
 written stations, **170ff**
Experiment, analytic, scoring of, **159** *Table 7.2*
Experiment station, skill assessment objectives of, **171**
Eye, use of in nonverbal communication, **62**
Eye examination skills, objectives of assessment of, **132**

Facial expressions
 in non-verbal communication, **63**
 showing emotions, **63** *Figure 4.2*
Feelings, ideas, function, and expectations, in assessing patient's concern, **76**
FIFE, *see Feelings, ideas, function, and expectations*
Focus question, use of, **202**
Format of questions at
 a structured viva, **202**
 a written station, **181**
Formative assessment, of trainees, **5**

Gait examination, assessing skills of, **130**
Griev_ing, model for
 assessing communication skills, **68**
 breaking death news, **68**
 death notification, **68**

Hands, uses of, in nonverbal communication, **61, 80**
Happiness, facial expression showing, **63** *Figure 4.2*
Harden, Ronald, OSCE founder, **10**
Hearing difficulty, assessment of, **133**
Hints and tips, for candidates, at
 communication skills stations, **76**
 OSPE stations, **170**
 physical examination stations, **102**
History- taking
 competencies assessable at, 38
 components and functions of, **30**
 contents and process of, **37**
 peculiarities of, in OSCE, **30**
 recording and presenting findings of, **37**
 techniques, **33ff**
History-taking skills, assessment criteria in PACES, **228** *Table 10.2*
History- taking stations, **47ff**
 abdominal pain due to ectopic pregnancy, **51**
 breathlessness, **53**
 competencies expected of candidates at, **33**
 examples of, **50ff**
 pain due to acute pancreatitis, **50**
Hypertension, counselling on management of, **85**

Imaging test materials, at a Written Station, **183ff,** *Figure 8.2*

Instruments and devices
 at a *viva voce* station, **206191**
 at a written station, **18370**,
 at an examination stations, **984.** *See also Diagnostics*
 at a written station, **170** *Figure 8.1*
 in OSPE, **169**
Interpersonal and communication skills, definition of, **60**
Interview findings
 how to present, **38**
 how to record, **38**
Interview, contents of, **38**
Introductory question, in Structured Viva, **202**
Investigation, explanation of, to patient, **84**

Justice, ethical principle of, **60**

Kalamazoo Consensus, on Medical Communication, **68**

Listening skills, components of, **66**

Macy Initiative, in Communication Skills, **68**
Management plan skills, following clinical assessment, **104**
Marksheet examples of
 for written stations, **185ff**
 for structured viva voce, **210f,** *Table 9.2*
Model for skills assessment of
 basic life support, **158**
 history taking, **33f**
Medications
 dispensing skills, of, **175**
 refusal to take, counselling skills on, **82**
Microscopy skills, assessment of, **171**

INDEX

Miller, George, pyramid of
    competencies of, **4**
Mnemonics, examples
    CHLORIDE PP **34**
    OLD CARTS, **34**
    OPQRST, **34**
    SOCRATES, **34**
    history taking , **34**
    initiating physical
        examination, **103**
Model answers, to sample questions
    for a structured viva station, **210**
    for written stations, **187ff**
Models of communicating bad news,
    ABCDE, **68**
    GRIEV_ING, **68**
    S-P-I-K-E-S, **68**
    SEGUE, **68**

Neurological examination skills, lower
    limbs, assessment of, **129**
Nonmaleficence, ethical principle
    of, **60**
Non-verbal communication
    examples of, **61, passim,** *Figures 4.1 and 4.2*
    interpretation of, **61, 80f**

Objective Structured Clinical
    Examination
    behaviour at , **25f**
    dress code for , **25**
    key features of , **14**
    station, operational elements at, **22**
    structure and purpose of, **11**
    tips and hints, for candidate
        during, **22ff**
Objective Structured Practical
    Examination
    assessable skills at, **165**
    circuit, schematic, **166,** *Figure 7.1*
    features of, **167**
    functions and uses of, **165**
    instruments and devices, for
        testing candidates at, **169f**
    stations, examples of, **170ff**
    test materials at, **169,** *Figure 7.2*
    types of, **164**
Operational elements at
    OSCE stations, **22**
    OSPE stations, **168**
    Practical procedure stations, **139**
    Written stations, **181**
Oral examinations, advice to
    candidates on , **212**
Orals, traditional, merits and demerits
    of, **199,** *Table 9.1*
OSCE stations, test materials at, **23,** *Table 2.3*
OSCE, see Objective Structured
    Clinical Examination
OSCE, variants of, **14**
OSLER, see variants of OSCE
OSPE, see variants of OSCE
OSPRE, see variants of OSCE
Oxygen therapy, rating objectives
    of, **154**

Pain
    abdominal
        due to ectopic pregnancy, **51f**
        due to pancreatitis, **50**
        scoring system for, **47**
    assessment of
        history taking, objectives of , **50**
        using the mnemonic
            SOCRATES, **34**
        skills at taking history of, **42,** *Table 3.1*
Patient education
    on use of PEFR, **90**
    techniques of, **80**

Patient, standardised history for,
example of, **39**
Patient concerns,
assessing skills at exploration of
, **230**
assessment of, **76**
Patient's history, stimulated, examples
of, **45f, passim**
Peak Expiratory Flow Rate Meter,
educating patient on, **90**
Performance by candidates,
assessment of
factors affecting, **12** *Figure 2.2*
template for rating of, **114**
using checklist and rating scales
in, **21**
Peripheral arterial disease, assessment
objectives for, **128**
Physical examination
diagnostics for, **98,** *Figure 5.1*
in PACES, assessment criteria for,
233, *Table 10.5*
Physical examination skills
Abdominal, example of, **108**
criteria for assessment of, **231**
how to close the encounter, **104**
in an OSCE exercise, **103**
objectives of assessment of, **111**
Physical examination, approach
in OSCE, **22**
in PACES, **233**
Physical examination station
assessment domains, **105**
differences between routine and in
OSCE, **94**
objectives and functions of, **94**
Skills assessable at, **94**
themes, for testing of, **118**
Physical signs, that can be
mimicked, **96**
Positioning of doctor and patient

at history taking, **40**
during physical examination, **100f,**
Figure 5.1
Post-encounter stations, **193**
Posture, in nonverbal communication,
80, passim
Potential tasks for Structured Oral
Examination, **216**
Practical Assessment of Clinical
Examination Skills (PACES)
and OSCE, compared, **228**
attributes of a good performance
at, **234**
overview of, **222ff**
structure of, **224,** *Figure 10.1*
Practical Procedure Skills Station,
categories of, **138**
examples of test materials at, **141**
frequently featured tests, **142f**
types of, **141**
Practical procedures, common
instruments and devices at, **141,**
Figure 6.1
Presenting complaint, common
examples of, **41f**
Procedures, explanations of, to
patients, **84ff**
Professionalism, testing of, **31**
Protocols, for clinical procedures
basic life support, **158**
history taking, **35**
recording clerking data, **36**
starting physical examination, **117**
Protocols, suitable for delivering bad
news
ABCDE, **68**
GRIEV_ING, **68**
S-P-I-K-E-S, **68**
Pyramid of competencies, Miller's,
3,6, *Figure 1.1*

INDEX

Questioning skills, in effective communication, **64**

Rating scale, use of
   in assessing candidate performance, **21**
   in assessing skills of blood pressure measurement, **136**
Respiratory system, objectives of physical examination of, **146**

Sadness, facial expression of, **61, 63,** *Figure 4.2*
Scoring system in PACES, **228**
Seating position, during history-taking, **43,** *Figure 3.1*
SEGUE, model for delivery of bad news, **68**
Skills, examinable, at physical examination station, **105**
Skin, objectives of examination of, **134**
Static or written station
   advice to candidates on, **183**
   common test materials at, **183**
   model answers to sample questions at, **183ff**
SOCRATES, as a mnemonic for pain history, **34**
Standardised patient, briefing, **45ff;** *See also simulated patient*
Station activities, in PACES, **228,** *Table 10.1*
Station, in performance-based assessment
   couplet, **18**
   manned and unmanned, **18**
   numbers and types in OSCE, **17,** *Table 2.1*
   number and types in PACES, **226**
   rest, **17**

Steroid therapy, objectives of station on, **86**
Structure, schematic, of
   OSCE, **11**
   OSPE, **166,** *Figure 7.1*
   PACES, **224,** *Figure 10.1*
Structured *viva voce* Station
   format of, **206**
   merits and demerits of, **199**
   model answers to sample questions at, **121**
   question types at, **207192**
   Structured *viva voce*, materials for, **206,** *Figure 9.2*
   tasks, examples of, **201ff**
Subjective and Objective (findings), Assessment, and Plan
   SOAP, acronym for record keeping technique, **37**
   use of, in approach to planning management, **104**
Summative assessment, of trainees, **5**
Symptom, attributes or dimensions of, **34**

Tasks, assessable at OSCE stations
   common examples of, **19,** *Table 2.1*
   viva, structured, examples of, **207ff**
   written examples of, **185**
Test materials
   for use at a Written Station, **182f**
   types of, at Structured Oral Examination Station, **206**
Tips and hints for candidates at
   history-taking station, **43**
   OSPE stations, **170**
   physical examination station, **102ff**
TOSCE, see variants of OSCE

Trainee assessment, types of, **5**
Triangulation, in trainee assessment, principles of, **6**
Tumour or mass, examination of, **136**

Veins, of lower limbs, examination of, **126f**
Verbal and non-verbal communications examples of, **57** *Figure 5.1*
Verbal communication, **61f**
Viva voce
    demerits and merits of, **199**

    traditional, purpose of **198**
    seating positions at, **203,** *Figure 9.1*
Vomiting, history of, assessment objectives on, **21,** *Table 2.2*

Written station
    examples of, **183ff**
    features of, **180**
    other names for, **180**
    purpose of, **180**

www.ingramcontent.com/pod-product-compliance
Lightning Source LLC
Chambersburg PA
CBHW020734180526
45163CB00001B/233